99

Anna Sproule

Whose Body is It?

E690 J/soc

Macdonald

A MACDONALD BOOK

© Anna Sproule, 1987

First published in Great Britain in 1987 by
Macdonald & Co. (Publishers) Ltd
London and Sydney
A BPCC plc company

ISBN 0 356 13410 5

Editor Donna Bailey
Production Controller Rosemary Bishop
Picture Research Diana Morris

Printed in Great Britain by
Purnell Book Production Ltd
Member of the BPCC Group

Macdonald & Co. (Publishers) Ltd
Greater London House
Hampstead Road
London NW1 7QX

BRITISH LIBRARY
CATALOGUING IN PUBLICATION DATA

Sproule, Anna
    Whose Body Is It?.—(Debates; 15).
    1. Health
    I. Title II. Series
    613   RA776
    ISBN 0-356-13410-5

Contents

It's my body,

Everyone has a body. Some would argue over whether it's their most precious possession, but all would agree that it is their most personal one. Your body is your machine for experiencing life.

You cannot live through someone else's body: if you are hungry, it is no good watching someone else eat the food you need. Unless you are an identical twin, no one even has a body that looks like yours, either. And even identical twins each have their own body, their own point of awareness, contained in a physical structure that can receive messages and transmit them, absorb material to fuel its activities, and carry out its owner's wishes.

A threat to our independence? Because they are so personal to us, we all care fiercely about things that happen to our bodies. They happen to *us* – not to anyone else. If someone else starts deciding what these things should be, we can experience a variety of unpleasant emotions: frustration, fear, anger. We would, for example, probably be angry at the way the other person is laying down the law about something that's not their affair. Our independence as individuals is threatened; our bodies are our uniquely personal business, and we alone should have the final say in what happens to them.

We might also experience pain – and, again, the pain happens to us, not to the person who is causing it. If someone causes us physical pain or harm, or forces us to cause pain to ourselves, we will react very strongly indeed. And we will have every right to do so.

A right to self-protection? Humans are social animals, and most humans live in social groups rather than in isolation. The societies they live in all seek to ensure their own survival as groups, and they do this by – among other things – laying down rules that promote social stability, prevent disorder and disruption, protect the weak, and ensure an optimum rate of population growth.

Very often, the rules affect what happens to our bodies. A society with a population problem, for example, will tend to make tough regulations about sex and birth control. A society that feels threatened could well lay much stress on deeply-dreaded physical punishments. A society trying to establish (or re-establish) its identity might have strong views on how its members appear to the outside world; how they behave, how they dress and so on.

In all cases, violent conflicts can arise. On one side are the people who feel that the social group is justified in protecting itself in these ways; on the other are those who feel their fundamental rights over their most personal possession are being eroded. The conflicts are often made even fiercer by the fact that people's ideas of what should or should not happen to our bodies are continually shifting. What's wrong in one setting may suddenly become right in another; what seems wrong to us may seem acceptable to our children.

So the battles are continually refought, on battlegrounds that continually change. This book describes some of them.

Opposite A French beach – or a battleground in the body ethics war? Until very recently, it was unthinkable for women to expose their breasts in public. But these sun-bathers would also cause a stir if they started going topless in the streets of their home towns. Notions of the right (or wrong) thing to do often depend strongly on where and when you do it.

> 'People have all sorts of taboos about their bodies.' Lord Avebury, announcing plans to bequeath his corpse to a dogs' home for food in 1987

> 'Being careful isn't just a personal precaution – it's a social responsibility as well.' Lindsay Shapero, writing in Company on safe sex, 1987

isn't it?

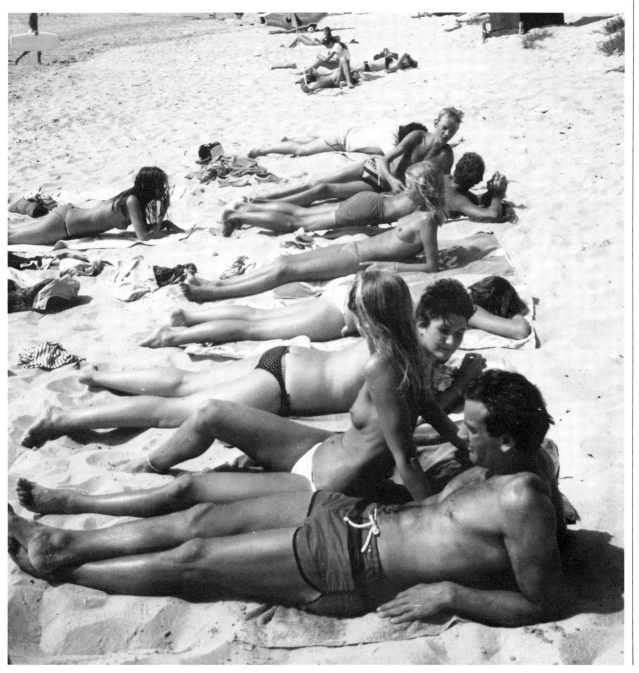

A question

I f we, as individuals, don't always control what happens to our bodies, who does? Very often, it's a doctor – or a great many doctors, whose research findings happen

to agree. Often again, it's the police. Or it might be a religious leader: either a leader of the religion we believe in, or that of the majority of people in our society. Many countries use the police to help ensure we stay in physical health; in some, the police force makes sure we stay in spiritual health as well. Teachers are yet another group that have a role to play in deciding how we should use our bodies. And parents make up the biggest group of all.

All these people are authority figures in our lives. To a greater or lesser extent, society gives them the right to dictate how we should behave. It also gives them powers to force us to do what they say. But, although we may have to go along with these decisions, we do not have to accept that they are necessarily good ones – or good ones for us. To make up our minds, we need to examine the motives of the people who make them. We also need to examine the skills they bring to the job.

Good advice? Imagine that, on a holiday abroad, you are about to try some new food of wildly exotic appearance. You are in a group with some relations, some friends, and someone who belongs to the country you are in. This person has ordered the dish, too – but points out that some

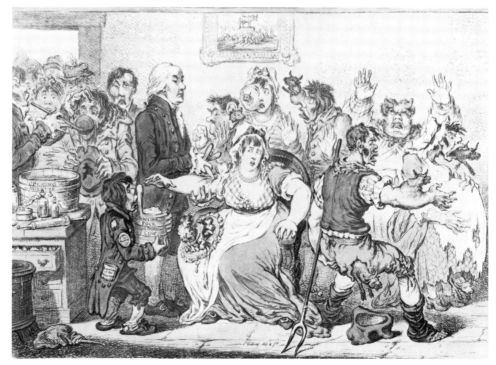

Some people trust doctors; others – as indicated by this cartoon of 1802 – do not! In fact, the doctor shown here is trying out one of the great life-saving techniques of medicine: vaccination against smallpox, using matter from a cowpox sore as a vaccine. So was the cartoonist's attack justified?

# of trust?

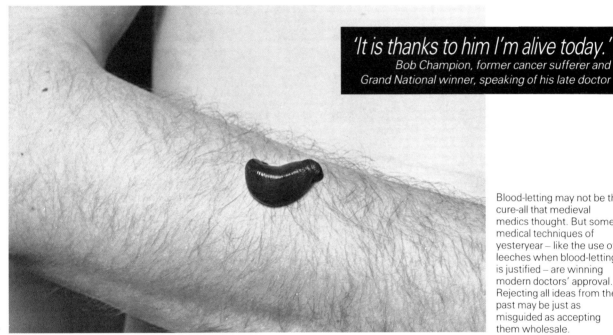

Blood-letting may not be the cure-all that medieval medics thought. But some medical techniques of yesteryear – like the use of leeches when blood-letting is justified – are winning modern doctors' approval. Rejecting all ideas from the past may be just as misguided as accepting them wholesale.

foreigners don't like it. Your relatives are worried that it might disagree with you. Your friends think you're mad, but urge you to carry on.

Your relatives have your best interests at heart. Your friends understand your adventurous nature. The foreign national has seen it all before. Which one is giving you the best advice? How far do motives contribute to its value, and how far does knowledge?

Sound fact – or nonsense? The trouble with well-meaning advice is that it is often based on insufficient knowledge. The doctors of the Middle Ages swore by blood-letting for all manner of ills, from deafness to indigestion. Today, we know that is nonsense.

There may be flaws in the adviser's motivation, as well: in the 19th century, many sincerely religious people (doctors in-

cluded) rejected the newly-developed use of anaesthetics for mothers in childbirth. The Bible, they pointed out, had said 'In sorrow thou shalt bring forth children.' It took no less a person than Queen Victoria, by then mother of seven, to make them drop this argument. Which did these doctors really find more important: their personal morality or the welfare of the women they were treating?

No position to judge? However, there's another problem still. Often we are in no position to judge the extent of an authority figure's knowledge, because we lack it ourselves. That is why we may be seeking advice in the first place. So, in the end, deciding whether someone's decision is a good one for us may come down to deciding how far we trust them. Or is it a matter of deciding how far they have earned our trust?

The best way to learn?

Opposite (top) After a beating: the boy's buttocks clearly show the extent of the injuries inflicted on him. Corporal punishment is now banned in British state-run schools, and private schools are being advised to do the same. Beating a schoolchild without parental consent is condemned by European law.

From the beginnings of recorded history, parents in many societies have trained children how to behave by beating them. The beaters, who included teachers and employers as well as parents, often inflicted severe injuries on the beaten; some children were even beaten to death.

Even today, many adults in the western world can remember seeing corporal punishment used at school (even if it wasn't used on them). And almost everyone has been smacked by their parents. But corporal punishment in schools is now becoming much less common than it was; in Britain, for example, state-run schools stopped using it in 1987. However, British private schools – including the famous 'public' ones – can still go on using the cane. So, as a result, will the arguments go on about whether it is right to train children by means of hurting their bodies.

A short, sharp shock? Any parent of an inquisitive, lively toddler will say that there are times when only a smack will do. These times come when, for example, the toddler is about to grasp something like a carving knife or the cat's tail. The smack is a 'short, sharp shock': it breaks the situation, snatches the toddler out of imminent danger, and rams the lesson home, all in one.

Taken into the school setting, the 'short, sharp shock' of a beating – along with the drama that surrounds it – can again break up a disciplinary situation that is getting out of hand. Especially when, as is usual, it is reserved as the ultimate deterrent, it also forces the lesson home like nothing else can. And many who have had the cane say that, while it certainly hurt, it didn't do them any harm in the long run.

Don't rewards work better? Opponents of corporal punishment say that fear does not breed the right conditions for learning anything, from maths or cookery to acceptable behaviour. At all levels, the best teaching strategy is one that puts the main stress on rewarding good behaviour rather than punishing bad. They also point out that the British experiment with 'short, sharp shock treatment' for young offenders (a short period of strictly-disciplined detention) appears to have failed.

In addition, classroom beatings, far from cowing wrong-doers, encourage the growth of a macho 'they can't scare me' code of behaviour that doesn't help learning either. And can it ever be right to use violence for any reason against a defenceless (and often very much smaller) opponent? What starts as a smacking has too often been known to turn into full-scale assault, leading to permanent physical and mental scarring.

> 'Through your counsel you said the merit of corporal punishment is that it is quick and hurts at the time, and is soon over and forgotten. I don't accept that this beating would be forgotten by this boy in his lifetime.'
> British judge Peter Crocker, sentencing headmaster to jail for causing actual bodily harm to pupils

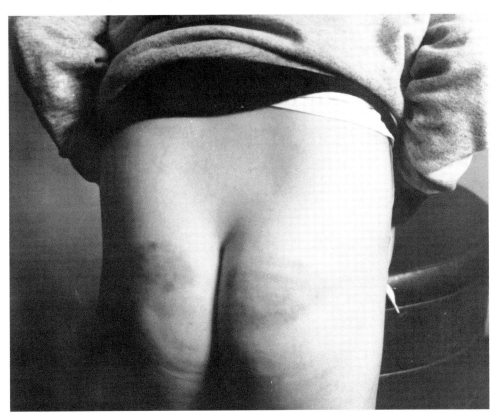

Below Corporal punishment used to be unquestioningly accepted as a way of enforcing discipline on young people, both in and out of school. The caption originally published with this engraving of 1831 summed up the reason: 'He that chastiseth one, amendeth many.'

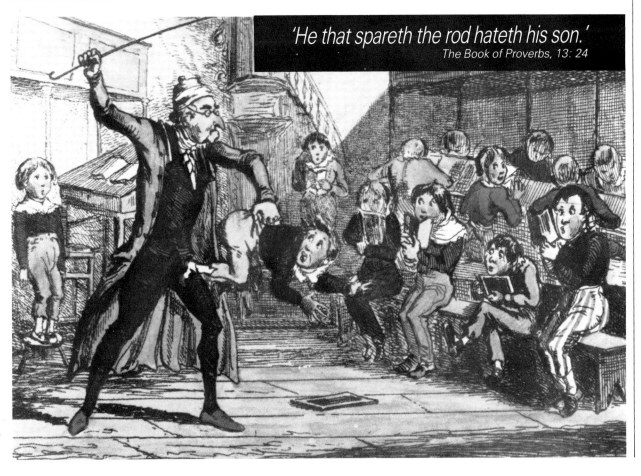

'He that spareth the rod hateth his son.'
The Book of Proverbs, 13: 24

A private affair?

Almost every culture has strong feelings and rules about one of the most private activities of human life: sexual intercourse. In fact, the idea that sexual intercourse should be a private thing, carried out away from the eyes of others, is one of the strongest rules of all, and probably an instinctive one. But there are many others; so many that they are often contradictory.

Given the world's huge variety of cultures, it's no surprise that a relationship that's encouraged in one place should be condemned in another. But how far should any society have the right to decide who goes to bed with whom?

So you think you own me? People who reject restrictions over sexual behaviour argue that most of these are based on the notion of a person's body being 'owned' by another person. According to traditional codes of conduct, people should only make love to the partners to whom they 'belong': their husbands or wives. However, the idea of owning someone else's body reduces that person to the status of little better than a slave.

In addition, the long-standing existence of 'ownership' rules has given all those who were brought up with them a deep sense of guilt about their bodies and bodily functions. The revolution that took place in

After the Liberation of France at the end of World War Two, women accused of sleeping with German soldiers had their heads shaved by furious patriots. Here, Parisian crowds hound a young woman suspected of collaboration. Note the expression of the Parisians' faces. Do they really express moral outrage?

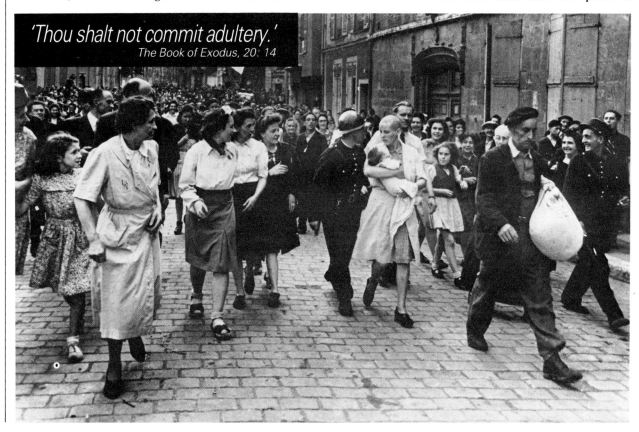

'Thou shalt not commit adultery.'
The Book of Exodus, 20: 14

the 1960s and 1970s against conventional sexual morality freed many people from a tangle of sex-linked emotions that harmed rather than helped them. Freeing sex from guilt allowed it to be put in its true perspective: a source of personal pleasure and release.

Another consequence of the '60s rebellion was that changes of sexual partner became much more socially acceptable than they had been. People who might have been condemned to a lifetime of unhappiness now had a chance of starting again in a fresh partnership. Meanwhile, efficient contraception was lifting the fear of long-term consequences from short-term sexual relationships.

What about the children? Opponents of sexual permissiveness stress that, whatever the intentions of the individuals involved, the biological purpose of sexual intercourse is to reproduce the species. Children need a stable, protective environment in which to develop, and many people think this is best provided in a traditional – and stable – marriage. Since it is in society's interests that its future members should develop well, society has a legitimate interest in promoting sexual fidelity rather than sexual experimentation.

Again, sexual intercourse can transmit several diseases, including AIDS. Society has a legitimate interest in ensuring the health of its members and thus has another reason for dictating sexual patterns, especially amongst young people, who may lack the experience to weigh dangers for themselves.

It can be argued, too, that young people can be damaged emotionally by sexual experimentation. In a permissive society, for instance, girls are often forced into reluctant sex by their boyfriends' expectations of them.

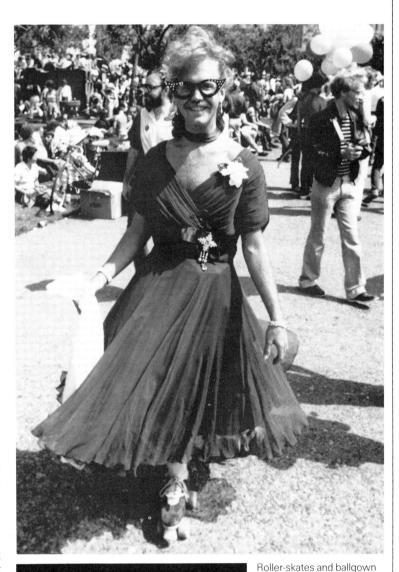

'Love can exist outside of marriage, and sex can certainly be an acceptable part of such a love.'
Dr C. H. Knickerbocker, 1968

Roller-skates and ballgown for a member of a Parade of Gays in San Francisco. Until recently, modern western culture strongly frowned on expressions of sexual love that focused on a partner of the same sex. Now, however, homosexuality has won widespread social acceptance, with California leading the way.

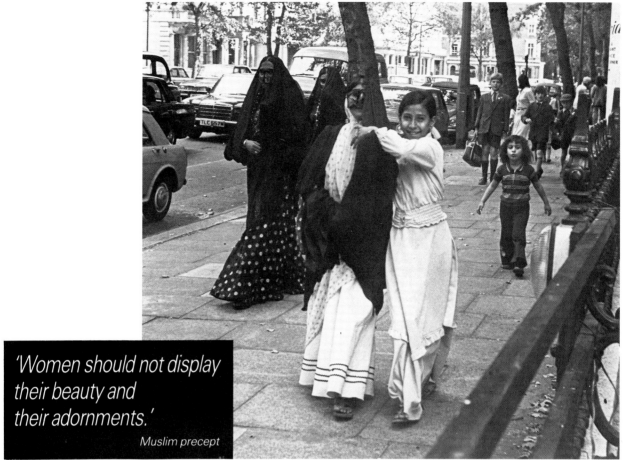

'Women should not display
their beauty and
their adornments.'

Muslim precept

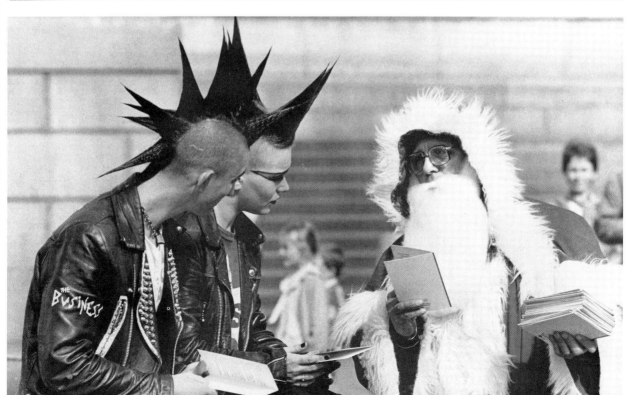

Style wars?

Schools hit the headlines for many reasons, serious and silly. One of the most enduring types of school story is also – according to some people – the silliest: the never-ending controversy over what constitutes a suitable school uniform. In fact, the strength of feeling aroused by these style wars shows that, in school and out, the issue of dress is for most people an extremely important one. Most of us have strong ideas of how we want to look. But, however we dress, there will always be someone who thinks we look totally unacceptable, and who wants to make us adopt their own views.

Right for the occasion? Many people would say that dress is first and foremost a practical matter. We wear clothes that are appropriate to our climate; we should also wear clothes that are appropriate to the occasion. In offices, for example, people are expected to work rather than to attract each other. Extreme fashions are therefore out. Jangling bracelets are out as well, since they drive other workers wild! People in schools are also meant to be working hard, so here, too, clothes are expected to be plain and sensible.

In addition, safety and health always have to be taken into account. In the Second World War, women workers poured into factories to make munitions. Their shoulder-length hair could have caught in the machinery, so they were urged to tie it up in headscarves; this then became a fashion in its own right. Today, doctors and parents frequently warn young people against the damage that can be caused by high-fashion shoes.

Employers, teachers, doctors and parents are all people who feel justified in dictating what other people should wear. So do religious leaders, who have the moral welfare of their congregations at heart. A special problem emerges here when religious symbols such as a cross are worn by obvious non-believers. People to whom the symbols are sacred have a case for feeling offended.

A means of self-expression? Most people would agree that there are some places and circumstances in which there must be rules governing dress. But they also point out that even uniforms soon get 'customized' to the extent that many of the basic aims of a uniform – safety, practicality and group cohesion – get lost. In Mao's China, for example, a whole society wore the 'Chairman Mao suit'. But the good cloth and tailoring that party bosses could afford were instantly recognizable.

Clothes offer people a legitimate method of self-expression, possibly one of the very few that are readily at everyone's disposal. Whether you have a little money or a lot, you can always make your clothes show how you feel about yourself, and how you want other people to feel about you. They are both a medium for creativity and an important system for social communication.

Opposite (top) Dress distinctions in a London street. The Arab women's cover-ups are in marked contrast with the cotton frock of the westerner in the background; so are the schoolboys' uniforms with the gear of the child in the T-shirt. The Arabs' dress is acceptable in Britain; would the clothes of westerners be acceptable in the Middle East?

Opposite (bottom) Meeting of extremes: London punks get Christmas cards from Santa Claus. Although both styles of dress seem wildly individual, both are in fact uniforms prescribed by tradition. The only real difference between them is that the punk tradition is newer.

> 'The turban is part of our faith and the Government cannot ask us to remove them.'
> Amar Singh Chhatwa, general secretary of the Sikh Cultural Society of Great Britain, on making safety hats compulsory wear on building sites

Laying down strict rules about clothes can also cause great dismay to groups with minority views. Sikhs, for instance, wear their turbans as part of their religion; efforts in Britain to introduce other kinds of headwear, such as safety helmets or crash helmets, have met with strong resistance.

The (slim) body

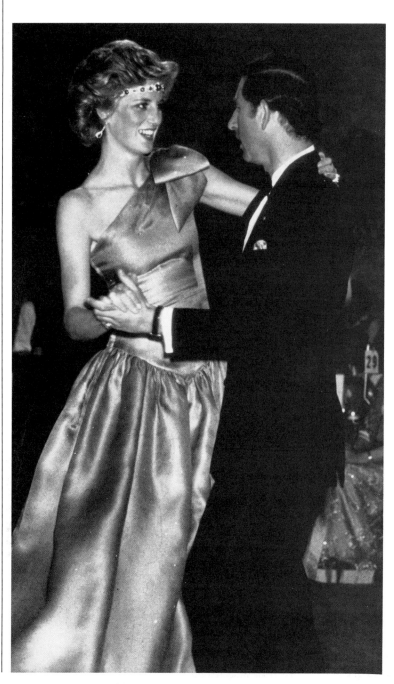

W here their bodies are concerned, women in the western world are today caught in a culture trap. When young, they are expected to be active, vital, slim and sexually attractive. When they grow older and acquire family responsibilities, this changes. They are now expected to be cuddly, nurturing, and 'mumsy', providers of warmth and home cooking. Research has shown, however, that married men would prefer their wives to go on being sexy and slim, even though this collides with the wives' new practical duties as nurturers.

Meanwhile, western society as a whole finds slim women of any age better-looking than fat ones. Although men also worry about their weight, a fat man has a better chance of being rated attractive than a plump woman. So weight worries are particularly a female problem, and one that often reduces women to misery. Does it make sense for them to worry?

Fatness can damage your health? In developed countries, where food intake is high and exercise output is often low, fatness is an endemic condition. High blood pressure and heart disease are also typical disorders in affluent western societies, and many doctors have pointed to a link between these and obesity. Fatness, in fact, can damage your health.

It can certainly also damage your social prospects. If society sees female obesity as bad, that's the way it is. Dieters would point out that, feminist arguments notwithstanding, they live in the real world rather than in an ideal one. In the real world, women who look good have a better, more rewarding life than those who don't. This applies to work, too: people who are rated physically attractive are thought to have other, less visible, virtues, such as intelligence and honesty.

beautiful?

On a practical level, the dieters would add, finding stylish clothes in large sizes is difficult – and, in a bikini, who wants to ripple about all over?

What's wrong with being big? Depressed dieters are often made even more dejected by the way many big eaters stay obstinately thin. In fact, doctors and nutritionists have started to question both the links between over-eating and obesity, and between obesity and illness. They also point to the ravages caused by the 'slimmers' disease', anorexia nervosa, which is very hard to treat.

Again, some experts feel that dieting, far from making you slim, will actually make you fatter in the long run. Dieters' bodies get used to functioning on less food. When the dieter reaches target weight and starts eating normally again, a lot more food is treated as fat-making 'surplus'.

'I don't regret a thing. It has given me a new lease of life.' Barbara Quelch, whose weight dropped by nearly half after an operation to halve the size of her stomach

'Being fat is not a big problem – people's attitudes can well be.' Carol Wilson, self-confessed 'large lady', 1986

More and more women are now consciously rejecting social commands to be slim, and learning to accept their bodies as they are. The reward, they say, is a big gain in self-confidence. Since self-confidence is the key to attractiveness, their decision to be big could actually help their social image much more than any obsession with getting thinner.

Opposite Idol of the western world, the Princess of Wales circles the ballroom in the arms of her husband. Diana's reed-like slimness is the envy of millions who long to copy her elegance.

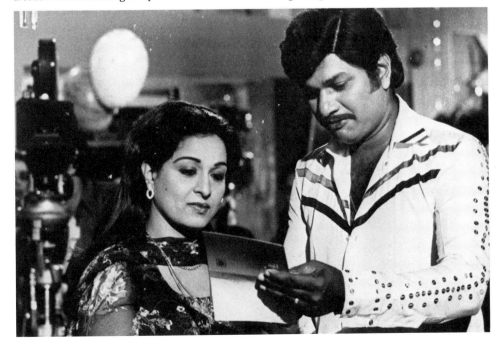

Leading Bangladeshi film stars Shabana and (right) Alam Gir demonstrate a different ideal of the body beautiful: plumper than the western one, but equally attractive.

Belt up and

D o we have the right to live danger-
ously? When, in the early 1980s, legal moves
were started in Britain to make people in
the front seats of cars wear safety belts,
controversy arose over just this point. A
common fear was that the British were
being overwhelmed by a 'Nanny State': a
benign, know-it-all entity that gently but
firmly deprived people of the opportunity
to do things that were bad for them.

The compulsory wearing of front-seat
safety belts is now accepted but, with the
wearing of backseat ones still optional, the
British continue to argue. Since few other
countries have followed the British example, the arguments are continuing elsewhere as well. Who is right: the safety
legislators or those who reject them?

An erosion of freedom? In a modern
society, the state already issues many
directions about how citizens should treat
their own and other people's bodies.
Ranging from building regulations about
nursery schools to rules about graveyards,
these directions are so all-embracing that
many people fiercely resist the idea of new
ones being added. The additions, they say,
are erosions of their freedom to run their
own lives and be responsible for their own
fate.

In the case of safety belts, they also point
to cases where victims of motor accidents
might have survived if they had not been
trapped in burning wreckage by belts that
they were unable to unfasten. In addition,
safety belts can be uncomfortable to wear,
especially if the wearer is pregnant or very
fat.

A further argument focuses on whether
safety belts are actually safe. Usually they
are only checked once a year at most, so
any faults or weaknesses that have developed may not be noticed until it is too late.

But the fact of having the belts in the car
will have meanwhile lulled those who rely
on them into a false sense of security.

What about the figures? The principal
argument in favour of safety belts comes
from motor accident statistics. The British
experience has shown that a drop in serious
accidents of between one-quarter and one-
third can be expected, following the introduction of legislation to make front seat-
belts compulsory. In the first year of compulsory seat-belt trials, the number of
serious accidents fell by 30 per cent. In the
two years following, the figures appeared
to drop less sharply. But, on the other
hand, the amount of traffic on the roads
had grown, so the decrease in the accident
rate had continued.

It is now accepted that motor accident
figures in Britain are at their lowest point in

Right Smoke belches from
wrecked vehicles in a
motorway pile-up. The fear
of being trapped in a blazing
car is one reason why people
are reluctant to wear safety-
belts.

Opposite Another aid to
drivers' safety: an inflatable
airbag that is normally
concealed in the hub of the
steering wheel, and inflates
if the car hits something at a
speed of 30 kph or over.

be saved?

30 years. Given a finding like this, many people would feel that a minor erosion of individual liberty is a small price to pay. They would also point out that the public expectations of what the state should do for its citizens have, over the last century, increased considerably.

Anyone, they say, who fears the effect of safety considerations on personal freedom is arguing like a Victorian supporter of *laissez faire* policy. This approach was summed up by a nineteenth-century report on industrial safety measures that said: 'It is a dangerous thing to liberty to have too much recourse to Government help to enable people to do what they are quite capable of performing for themselves.'

Today, however, people expect to live in conditions of safety – and they also expect the state to make sure those conditions exist.

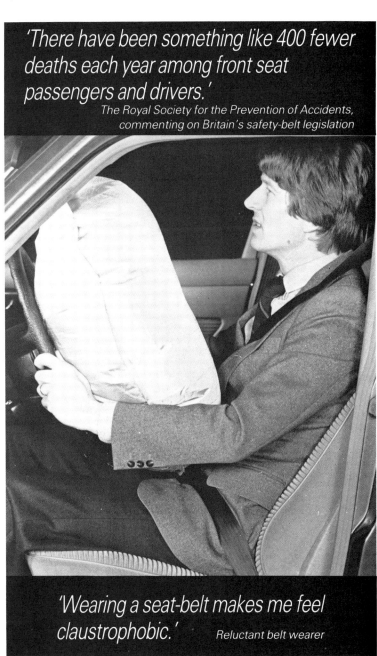

'There have been something like 400 fewer deaths each year among front seat passengers and drivers.'
The Royal Society for the Prevention of Accidents, commenting on Britain's safety-belt legislation

'Wearing a seat-belt makes me feel claustrophobic.' Reluctant belt wearer

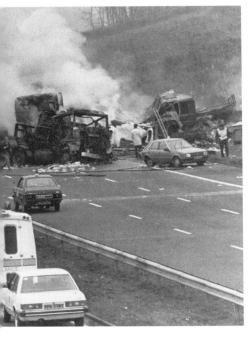

Thinking of

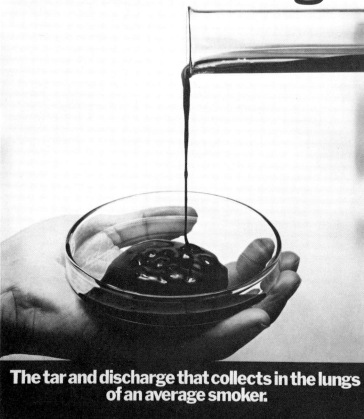

No wonder smokers cough.

The tar and discharge that collects in the lungs of an average smoker.

The Health Education Council

'Workers at a Chicago-based firm have been told never to smoke again, even at home, or be sacked. They will be forced to undergo lung tests to ensure compliance.'
The Times, *describing policy at USG Acoustical Products, 1987*

C igarette smoking has been enormously popular in the West for over a hundred years. Now, however, it looks as though it's on the way out as an accepted social habit. Although more young people are experimenting with cigarettes, more and more adults – especially men – are giving up. In Britain, for instance, only a third of the adult population now smokes; in the early 1970s, almost half did.

But many of those who have given cigarettes up will admit that it was a struggle. Meanwhile, many of those who do still smoke have tried to give up and failed. Should they think of trying again?

Helps you relax? People who defend the practice of smoking (they are usually, but not always, smokers themselves) point out that every society has its social drug. Nicotine is just one among many, and does less immediate widespread harm than, say, alcohol. Smoking a cigarette is not just a pleasant activity; it also helps the smoker either relax or concentrate, according to the occasion. Again according to the occasion, it is a useful medium for expressing messages about oneself: cigarettes fit both a macho image and an elegant, sophisticated one.

By giving smokers 'something to do with their hands', smoking eases the anxiety present in social situations. For those who are anxious even on their own, cigarette smoking is a way of structuring time: a smoker's daily pattern of consumption – one after breakfast, two on the drive to work and so on – can be a source of great reassurance in an unsettling world.

It is common to hear smokers say that the mere thought of giving up makes them so anxious they reach for a cigarette. They are less convinced than non-smokers of the link between smoking and disease, but point out that they have the right to risk

giving up?

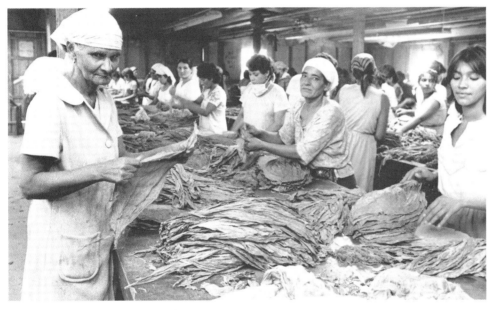

Nicotine is a popular drug, and many countries where tobacco grows easily have found that it is an important source of foreign earnings. If 'customer states' all banned smoking, these countries' incomes would fall dramatically – and what would happen to workers like these Nicaraguan women? Without tobacco production, there might be no jobs for them.

harming their own bodies. They can also all point to friends who have given up and then courted another health risk by putting on weight.

All preventable? Those who oppose smoking can produce much evidence to back their claim that smoking does not only endanger health; it kills. Doctors have calculated that the vast majority of people – ninety per cent – who die of lung cancer, chronic bronchitis and some other lung diseases do so because they smoked. Smoking is also linked with heart disease. Since smoking is a voluntary activity, these deaths are all preventable.

Although everyone has to die of something sometime, the evidence also points to the fact that smokers die younger than most non-smokers. On average, the life of a smoker is something like 12 years shorter than, statistically, it should have been. Almost half the people who smoke heavily do not even live long enough to retire.

You do not have to smoke, either, to run risks associated with smoking. Being exposed to other people's cigarette smoke turns you into a 'passive smoker'. On a car journey with a smoking driver, the passive smoker will be absorbing a third of each cigarette the driver smokes. If a pregnant woman smokes, she can damage the foetus in her womb.

Non-smokers also say that smoking – as a preventable cause of disease – wastes huge amounts of the money devoted to a society's health care; in Britain in 1984, the sum spent on smoking-related diseases was £170m. The same amount was therefore not available to spend on treating patients who had become ill through no fault of their own.

Opposite The power of the visual aid: one of the highly effective posters featured in the anti-smoking campaign of Britain's Health Education Council (now replaced by the Health Education Authority).

'Did I wake up in the Soviet Union this morning?'

Worker at USG in, 1987

It's my hangover,

In 1919, the United States of America became a 'dry' society: by an amendment to its national consitution, it outlawed alcoholic drink. All the same, however, Americans went on drinking and, in 1933, the amendment was repealed. US Prohibition had been a failure – mainly because it had proved unworkable.

However, it has not proved unworkable elsewhere. Muslim beliefs ban the use of alcohol, and many Muslim states are 'dry'. Other countries, Britain included, operate a partial sort of Prohibition through the restrictions they place on the sale of alcohol and the times at which it can be drunk in public.

Poorer without it? Both partial and total bans on drink attract huge amounts of criticism. The American version, in particular, won swift notoriety because of the way it actually made social conditions worse rather than better. By pushing drink underground, it turned the liquor business into something criminals could exploit. The result was the growth of nation-wide gangsterism.

Many people feel that heavy restrictions on drinking represent yet another attempt by the state to 'act the nanny'. Such restrictions, they say, interfere to an unacceptable extent with the liberty of the individual to decide his or her own conduct. They accept that alcohol can endanger health, but point out that drinkers have the right to choose whether to put themselves at risk. In moderation, they add, alcohol can even be good for you: many elderly people have been instructed by their doctors to have a regular glass of sherry or wine as a pick-me-up.

Furthermore, drinking alcohol is in itself an extremely pleasant activity. In the West, at least, it is also an all-pervasive one. From the family wedding to the quiet dinner party, from the business lunch to the session down the pub or club, alcohol underwrites social gatherings, gives a sparkle, provides an impetus. Western society would be the poorer without it.

It would be literally poorer as well, since the production of wine, beer and spirits forms an important element in many national economies. So do the taxes that can be levied on their purchase.

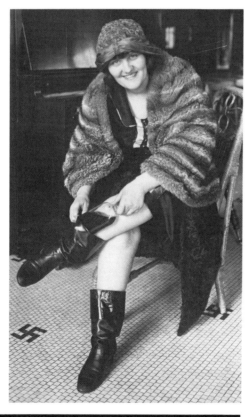

The not-so-grim face of American Prohibition: the ankle-flask in use. The original caption to this 1922 photograph read, 'Milady carries the dainty little silver trinket securely and safely tucked away in her Russian boot, fastened to the ankle, which may explain the sudden popularity of the boot, the newest thing in feminine footwear.' No-one seems bothered about the illegality of drinking the flask's contents – least of all its delighted owner!

'Drink no longer water, but use a little wine for thy stomach's sake and thine often infirmities.'

St Paul (I Timothy, 5: 23)

isn't it?

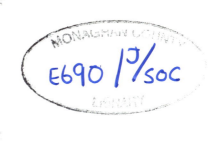

Too dangerous? Other people would argue that, pleasant as alcohol is, it is also a dangerous social drug: too dangerous to allow society to consume unhindered. Although – hangovers apart – moderate drinkers are at little physical risk from the practice, this is not true of heavy drinkers, who court the dangers of alcohol addiction, brain damage, and the killer disease cirrhosis of the liver.

However, the dangers to the individual drinker are only part of the picture. The dangers that his or her drinking habits pose to others are greater still. Even a small amount of alcohol makes a driver dangerous behind the wheel of a car, while a substantial proportion of crimes of violence – from football hooliganism to murder – are alcohol-linked.

> 'Why don't we see drink ads about people setting themselves on fire or crashing their cars or choking to death on vomit?'
> *Reformed teenage drinker, 1986*

Even where excessive drinking does not lead to violence, it can wreck the lives of drinkers and their families in other ways. It is an expensive habit to sustain. It can make the drinker unreliable at both work and home. The loss of a job will lead to additional money worries and further distress. Society has a right to be protected by law from the damage that alcohol can cause through the people who abuse it.

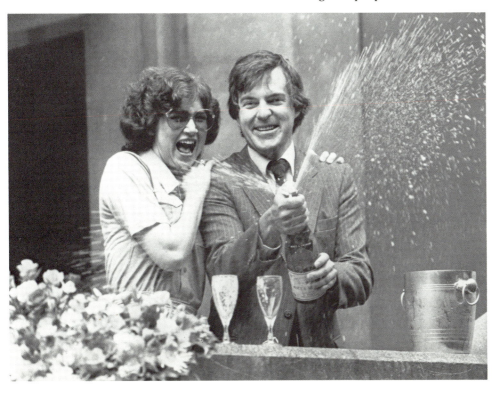

Giving a sparkle: without champagne, the celebrations for an engagement or wedding would seem woefully incomplete.

Babies of the state?

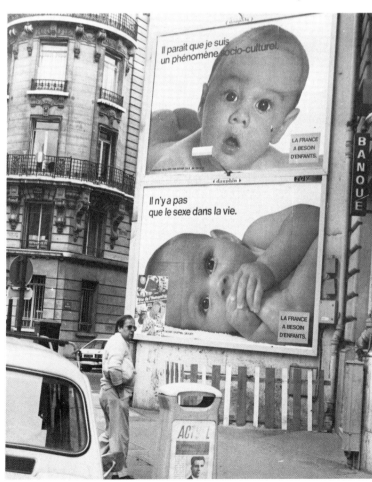

'It seems I am a socio-cultural phenomenon . . .' Enormous babies stare benignly down from hoardings all over France as part of a campaign to push the population up. 'France,' the posters add, 'needs children.'

Until fairly recently, the forces governing the growth or decline of a society's population were almost totally outside the individual's power to control. If there was a long period of peace and good harvests, people would have more to eat, female fertility would improve, more children would be born (and survive to have children themselves)... and the population would grow. But growth could readily be halted, even reversed, by great natural and man-made catastrophes such as famine, war and epidemics.

Too many people? A modern state has a legitimate interest in knowing how many people it has to cater for. Since it has to plan for the future, it has a further interest in knowing what the population trends are. In a country with an expanding population, how many new schools will need to be built? In a country with an ageing one, what is going to be done about increasing health care and money for pensions?

In both instances, the state has a problem to solve. To solve it, it may well want to manipulate the population trends that are the problem's cause. For some states, indeed, there is little room for argument. Modern China, for example, could face mass starvation in the fairly near future if its billion-strong population continues to grow at its expected rate. To save the nation, the Chinese have introduced a birth control policy that limits couples to one child each.

Finland has the opposite problem: a population that is already small and will soon get smaller. By next century, it will have dropped something like a million from its population of 4,900,000 and will have many more elderly people than it used to. Some Finns are suggesting the country should take in thousands of political refugees every year; others say that the government should encourage Finns to have more children. Across the border in the Soviet Union, many Russian couples voluntarily limit their families to one child, or remain childless; the government, which wants to push the numbers up, has put a special tax on childless couples.

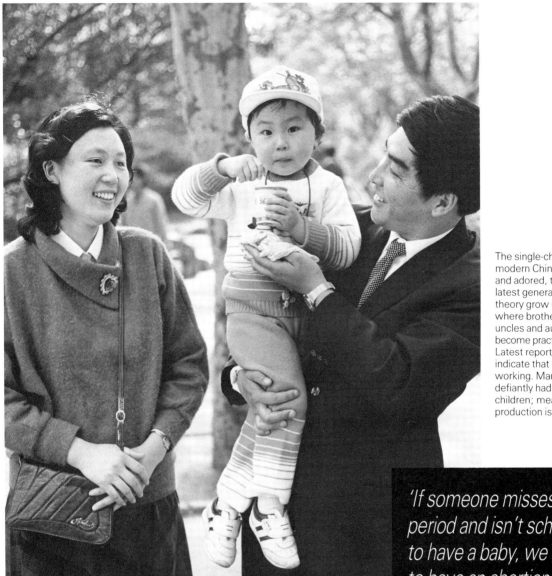

The single-child family of modern China: pampered and adored, the country's latest generation could in theory grow up into a culture where brothers, sisters, uncles and aunts soon become practically unknown. Latest reports, however, indicate that the policy is not working. Many Chinese have defiantly had second children; meanwhile, food production is falling.

'If someone misses her period and isn't scheduled to have a baby, we tell her to have an abortion.'
Chinese community warden, 1984

Aren't we the state? Many people would agree that the state has a duty to protect and provide for its people. But, they would add, the people *are* the state. What the state does should comply with their wishes, especially over a subject as personal as family size. If they want to remain childless on economic grounds, they should be allowed to. If – as in the Third World – they like to have large families for religious or cultural reasons, that should also be permitted.

Controversy also exists about the means used to enforce population control on unwilling populations. In India, for example, where the population problem is second only to China's, reports have circulated that in one state, the sterilization programme featured forced vasectomies. Furthermore, it's often argued that birth control programmes represent a western-style approach to the Third World's resource problems. Third World experts point out that these problems could be eased if the West used fewer resources itself.

'Be fruitful, and multiply, and replenish the earth and subdue it.' The Book of Genesis, 2: 28

In many parts of the world, couples who make love expect to use some contraception method as a matter of course. Elsewhere, however, such expectations are impossible: contraception methods are too expensive, too difficult to get, banned by church or state – or all three. Even in the affluent and permissive West, there are plenty of people who feel, for various reasons, that contraception is not for them. Their decision is often based on moral grounds, but so is that of the couples who do opt for birth control.

Why bear an unwanted child? Many who support contraception would argue that love-making really involves three people rather than two: the man, the woman and the child they may conceive. They point out that bringing up a child is a long, expensive and often challenging business, and the child's own chances of happiness are much increased if it is a wanted one. If, on the other hand, it is unwanted, it can face a future of haphazard parenting, material disadvantage and even abuse.

No child, the argument continues, should have to be born into conditions of outright deprivation. Couples should not be trapped by ignorance, poverty or religious or cultural demands into bearing children they cannot feed or house properly. Even if they are well-off, they should not be forced to have more children than they think their income and capabilities allow. And people who do not feel that they would make good parents certainly shouldn't be goaded into parenting.

Birth control is also desirable on health grounds. Couples who know they could pass a genetic disorder on to their children, should have the chance to opt for childlessness instead. Again, bearing too many children damages a woman's health – while some women may put their lives at risk if they only have one.

In the past, the practical demands of childbirth and caring for large families kept all but wealthy women confined to the life

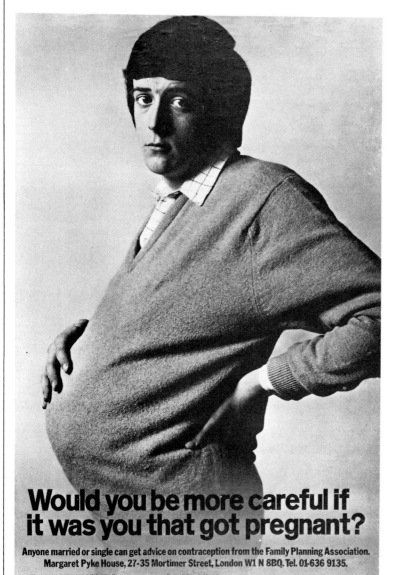

Would you be more careful if it was you that got pregnant?

Anyone married or single can get advice on contraception from the **Family Planning Association.**
Margaret Pyke House, 27-35 Mortimer Street, London W1 N 8BQ. Tel. 01-636 9135.

The Health Education Council

# of love ?

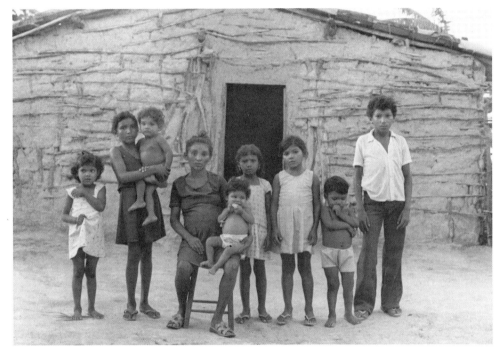

Dominated by her fertility, this Brazilian widow is only 30. Of her eight children, two are paralysed; a ninth is on the way.

of the home. Now that women can choose when (or if) to have children, they have the chance to explore their other abilities by taking jobs or careers. This may in the end raise their notoriously low social status.

Is it a sin? Many religious people, especially Roman Catholics, think most forms of birth control are sinful. Sin has to do with intentions as well as with acts. Preventing a sperm from fertilizing an ovum is wrong because it frustrates the natural purpose of the sex act: creating a new life. For this reason, contraception flouts the will of God.

The main contraception method Catholicism allows is abstinence: refraining from sex at times when women are most likely to conceive. Usually, religious people feel that abstinence or chastity – refraining from making love with anyone except a marriage partner – is good in itself. Historically, fear of pregnancy has helped enforce chastity, so anything that removes that fear is less than welcome. It is pointed out, too, that some contraception methods can damage women's health.

Again, in Third World countries, children are often looked upon as a source of wealth and support rather than a liability. A family with many sons can do more heavy work and grow more food; in old age, the parents will have someone to support them. They would therefore reject birth control on practical grounds.

> '*Only two? Oh, I'm so sorry, Madam.*'
> *Nigerian father of ten to Western mother of two*
>
> '*Pope denounces state aid for birth control.*'
> *Headline in* The Times, *November 1986*

So you're

Opposite According to a United Nations survey, over 80 per cent of all the births that take place in the western hemisphere in the year 2000 will probably be in Latin America. Against this prospect – and against the prospect of deprivation and poverty that it implies – the contraceptive pill gives these young Colombian women the chance to control their futures.

More than any other method of contraception, the contraceptive pill has revolutionized women's control over their own bodies. After it came into general use, women could rest almost totally assured that they would not become pregnant unless they wanted to. It seems no co-incidence that the spread of the women's liberation movement in the 1970s coincided with its arrival.

In spite of this, many women have now rejected the chance the pill offers them to

> 'But I don't want to be sterilized.' *Pill-user, aged 38*

take charge of the way their fertility works, when they want and as they want. Even before the AIDS epidemic brought the male sheath back into favour, sexually active women were changing back to other contraception methods. Many, too, found their only real alternative to the pill was the permanent contraceptive of sterilization.

Who'd deny its value? Few women would deny that the pill is the easiest and most convenient contraceptive to use. Very importantly, too, it places the responsibility for parenthood or the reverse squarely on the woman herself – which is where most of its users would wish it to be. It has the desirable side-effect of abolishing heavy or irregular menstruation. And there is no

argument over the fact that, properly taken, it is almost 100 per cent effective.

In addition, taking the pill can be actually safer than having a baby. In the United Kingdom, for instance, nine women out of every 100,000 die each year as a result of pregnancy and childbirth – a considerably higher figure than the one for young women who take the pill (and do not smoke).

How dangerous is it? As more and more women took the pill, doctors and scientists became increasingly alarmed. They observed it was appearing to have a wide range of side-effects that, far from being beneficial, were unpleasant and even dangerous. The milder ones included – for some women, though not all – weight gain and loss of sex drive. More serious were migraines, depression and moodiness that could swing into violence. More serious still was the link between the pill and blood clots. Doctors started putting women on the mini-pill, with its lower dose of hormones; they also began to warn pill-takers of over 35 to change to another method of contraception, especially if they smoked. In 1983, research started to point to the most fearsome link of all: between the pill and cancer of the breast and cervix. However, this link has not been proved.

Did the media help? No one would query a doctor's responsibility to warn a patient against the pill if it appeared to be potentially bad for her. No one, either, would

on the pill?

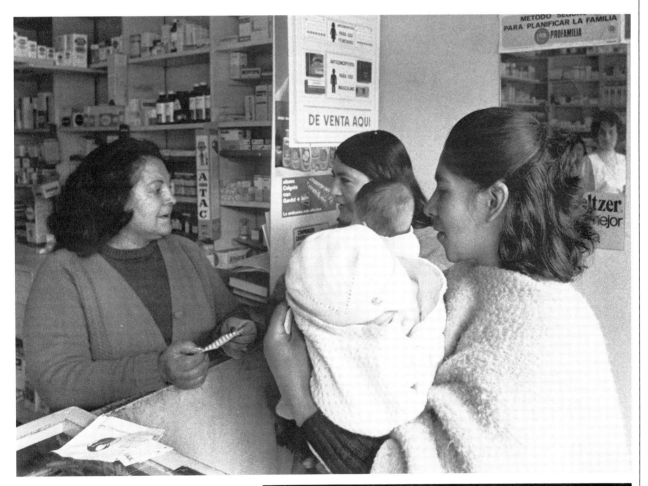

query researchers' rights to publish their findings, however much these upset people. But many would strongly criticize the role the media have played in turning these findings into 'scare stories' about the pill – with highly questionable results. After the cancer scare, for example, the abortion rate among young women shot upwards.

'It is often far from easy to make those "responsible decisions" family planning clinics urge upon us.'

Madeleine Kingsley, 1986

Mother knows best?

When a woman decides to have a baby, she embarks on life's most intimate relationship. For nine months, she carries another living person inside her body. For much of that time, the person-to-be could not survive without her. It absorbs the food she eats and the air she breathes; if her body is harmed or injured, it may suffer too.

Most societies have special rules and regulations that govern a woman's life when she is pregnant. In developed countries today, many of these focus on protecting the growing foetus's health. Often, though, they can conflict quite drastically with the mother's wishes – and sometimes with her rights.

Exposed to risk? If a mother-to-be smokes, her baby may be born smaller than average. If she has an alcoholic drink, the baby is affected by the alcohol. If she takes a medical drug, this too can affect the foetus, as is shown by the tragic international community of now-adult 'thalidomide children'. If she is hooked on a drug of addiction, her baby will be born a junkie. And if she has AIDS, the baby could well carry the virus too.

Obviously, the mother may expose herself to some of these risks by accident. But drug companies are now careful about potential risks to the unborn child, while everyone knows if he or she is having a drink, a smoke, or a fix. Most people know, too, that these things can injure the growing foetus.

So it can be argued that a mother who ignores the fact that such actions are dangerous is willingly endangering her child – and could therefore be breaking the law. Indeed, recent legal judgements in Britain and the USA have gone against a drug-addicted mother and one who, while also carrying her child, did not go to hospital when she was told to.

Is she really guilty? It can also be argued, however, that it is difficult to the point of impossibility to judge a woman's 'guilt' in the matter of her treatment of her unborn child. What if a treatment that (possibly) threatens the foetus is the only one that can save her own life? What about all the foetuses that *aren't* damaged by smoking or drinking? Given that these do exist, should smoking or drinking be made a crime for mothers-to-be?

Again, now that the law has acknowledged the concept of maternal liability, what will happen if children start sueing their mothers for ill-treatment? Only doctors and other professionals can really testify on this point, so will women who smoke or take drugs refuse to go to the doctor when they get pregnant?

Does the doctor know best? A similar problem surfaces when the time is come for the child to be born. In a doctor's judgement, the safest place to be born is a hospital, with advanced technology on hand in the event of an emergency. Many women, however, prefer to give birth at home, where the emotional and social aspects of childbirth are not outweighed by the medical ones. But supposing something goes wrong and the baby is harmed?

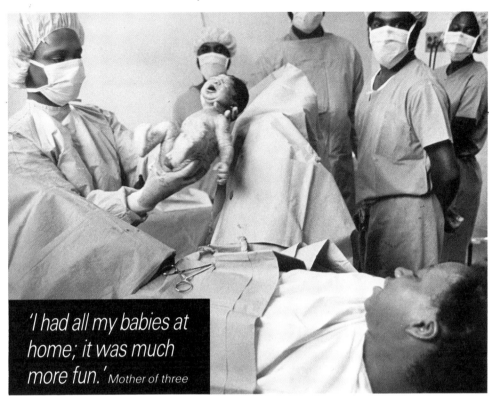

'I had all my babies at home; it was much more fun.' *Mother of three*

A mother beams, and a new-born child shrieks as it is brought into the harsh light of day. However efficient and devoted the care provided at a modern hospital birth, some people feel it is unneccessarily traumatic for both mother and baby: too clinical, too noisy, too impersonal.

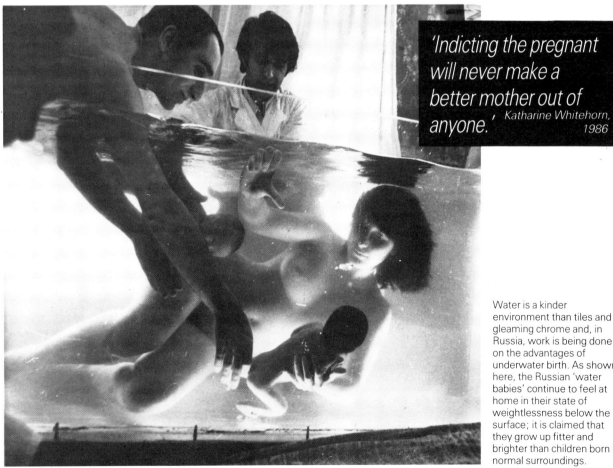

'Indicting the pregnant will never make a better mother out of anyone.' *Katharine Whitehorn, 1986*

Water is a kinder environment than tiles and gleaming chrome and, in Russia, work is being done on the advantages of underwater birth. As shown here, the Russian 'water babies' continue to feel at home in their state of weightlessness below the surface; it is claimed that they grow up fitter and brighter than children born in normal surroundings.

Abortion: the

Abortion is one of the oldest methods of controlling human fertility. In some countries, such as Russia, it is still used very frequently. In the West, its use was made legal only recently, in the wake of the social liberalization that took place in the 1960s. Even then, however, the idea of legal abortion was hotly attacked. These attacks have continued and, with the growing social reaction against '60s permissiveness, they now look likely to increase.

Can murder be condoned? Opponents of abortion say that, quite simply, abortion is murder. The foetus is both human and alive. It therefore deserves the protection society accords to all living humans. The fact that it is wholly at the mercy of others should merely deepen the responsibility that society feels towards its future members.

Some anti-abortionists are willing to stretch a point in cases where the decision presents a harsh and simple choice between the mother's life or the child's. Present western laws, however, permit abortions on grounds that are less black-and-white, such as risk to the mother's mental health. Such elasticity, anti-abortionists feel, cloaks many cases of 'abortion on demand': the murder of a future human on the whim of its present host. They also point out that abortion can be dangerous to the mother, even when carried out under clinical conditions. Some women have died under abortions, while others find their future fertility impaired, or suffer severe psychological damage.

What about the father? A further argument arises over the rights of the foetus's father. Suppose he wants the baby and his wife or partner does not? As things stand currently, he has no legal way of preventing the abortion of his child. In 1987, for example, British courts ruled against a father who tried to stop the mother of his unborn child having an abortion. However, Robert Herzc, a Norwegian father-not-to-be, has decided to test the issue of father's rights in the European Court of Human Rights.

How does the mother feel? Supporters of abortion point to the essential (and lengthy) part played in the development of the foetus by its mother. Since she is the other partner in the exercise, she too has rights that should be taken into account. And the first of these is the right to decide what should happen in her own body. If she does not want to have the child she has conceived – if its birth would damage her health, if she cannot afford to bring it up, if she feels unprepared for motherhood, if

Nurses and a priest join other British anti-abortion marchers in a demonstration in London's Piccadilly.

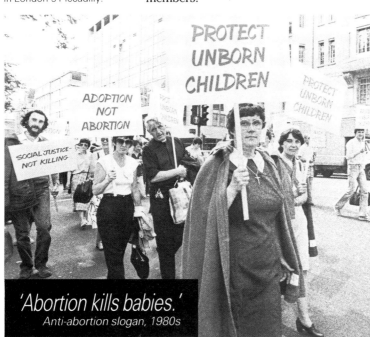

'Abortion kills babies.'
Anti-abortion slogan, 1980s

right to decide?

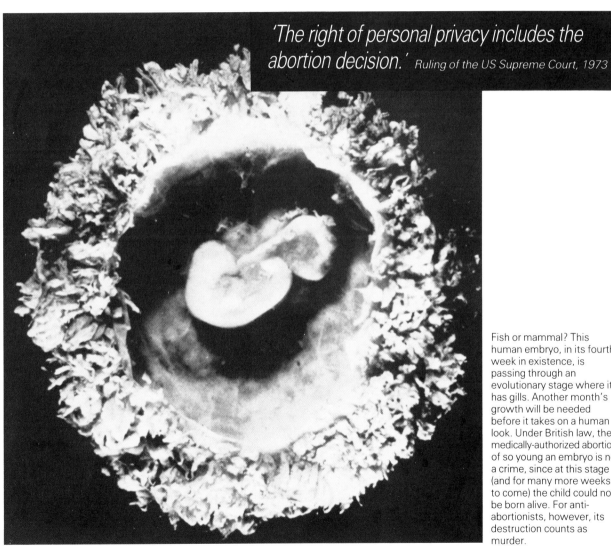

'The right of personal privacy includes the abortion decision.' *Ruling of the US Supreme Court, 1973*

Fish or mammal? This human embryo, in its fourth week in existence, is passing through an evolutionary stage where it has gills. Another month's growth will be needed before it takes on a human look. Under British law, the medically-authorized abortion of so young an embryo is not a crime, since at this stage (and for many more weeks to come) the child could not be born alive. For anti-abortionists, however, its destruction counts as murder.

she has been raped – she is entitled to bring the pregnancy to an end.

If it seems that the baby will be born with severe disabilities, then abortion is also justified – this time on the grounds of its own welfare. Indeed, pro-abortionists would argue, who has the right to condemn a human to a life of exceptional difficulty and pain, if it is known in advance that this is likely?

On the safety factor, they would add that the safety record of legal abortions is improving – and that nothing could be as dangerous to the mother's health as the old 'back-street' abortion performed in conditions of secrecy and squalor.

The forbidden frontier?

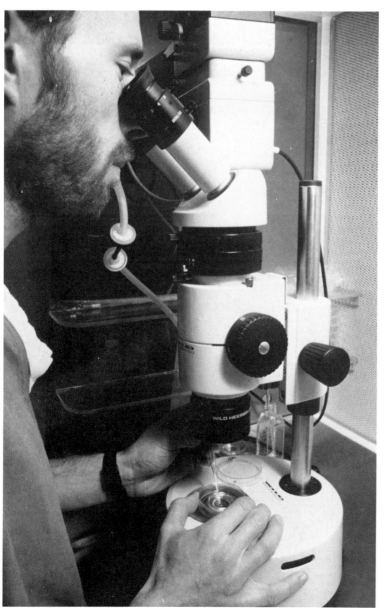

Doctors and scientists have recently made huge strides in developing techniques for working with the human embryo before birth. Embryos can now be created outside the womb – some becoming the famous 'test tube babies' – and operated on inside it. As more and more possibilities for work on the embryo open up, people have become increasingly worried. Are the scientists beginning to go too far? Is their work taking them towards a sort of forbidden frontier, beyond which no one should venture?

Why hold back? The aim of all researchers, medical or not, is to acquire more knowledge. Most would react with incomprehension to the idea that they should refrain in principle from pushing back the barriers of ignorance. Research on the human body in its earliest stages of existence can open up areas of knowledge whose value can only be guessed at. If such research were banned, scientists would have problems like those faced by doctors in the Middle Ages, when the Church vetoed the dissection of human bodies.

Obvious ways in which embryo research might help society include the study of infertility (a cause of enormous distress to many couples), contraception, and the correction of genetic abnormalities. If the genes that cause genetic defects can be isolated, this is an enormous step forward to abolishing the defect itself. Research on the pre-birth body is an important part of genetic exploration.

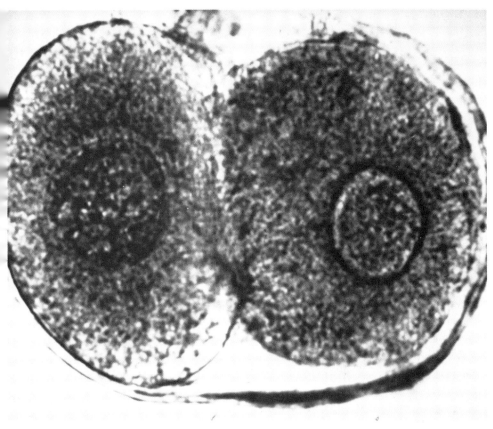

The beginning of life: 60 hours after it is fertilized by a sperm, a human ovum performs its first cell division. It is now an embryo.

Embryo researchers accept there have to be controls on their work. Many voluntarily impose their own, like outlawing cloning (using a portion of a parent organism to grow an identical copy), genetic manipulation and all work on an embryo, or 'pre-embryo', that's older than 14 days. Pre-embryos are sometimes grown on purpose from eggs given for research by women being sterilized; others are 'spares' from the test-tube baby process.

Cold-blooded? Many people believe that, even at 14 days old or younger, the embryo is a living human body that deserves the legal protection given to all humans. Using it for research work, then discarding it, is tantamount to using and discarding a person; it is damaging God's creation and murdering a human in a particularly cold-blooded way.

It is also often pointed out that scientists have a responsibility to humanity that goes beyond the mere accumulation of knowledge. The researchers of today have no real control over what will be done with their work in the future; if they feel they are making discoveries that could be grossly misused, they have a duty to call their work to a halt.

What really frightens people about embryo research is the possibility it could open up for manipulating genes to create 'humans to order'. From there, it would be a short step to the nightmares now only envisioned by science fiction: master races, slave classes, human breeding programmes and the rest. Although this sounds far-fetched, the scientific realities of today would have seemed equally unlikely to our great-grandparents. Today's research blessing for mankind could well, it is feared, turn into tomorrow's curse.

Opposite IVF in progress. In an ultra-clean environment, and using a microscope, a technician monitors events in a glass Petri dish – the 'vitro' of the technique's name. Sperm have just been added to the ova the dish holds.

'Without this research going on we would be childless.'
Father of 'test-tube' baby in, 1986

'The idea of the male pregnancy is not entirely new. Initial research was conducted in the 1960s on mice . . . with the minute embryo growing in the anterior chamber of the eye.'
Robin Kent, on the possibility of the male pregnancy, 1986

Keeping it in

Although, in the West, sex education of some sort is now an established part of the programme in many schools, the controversy it has always attracted continues as strongly as ever. Indeed, with the arrival of AIDS, it has probably grown even stronger. Is school the right place for teaching young people how to deal with their own sexuality?

What will it lead to? For many people (and especially for parents) it is difficult to accept the idea of children as sexual beings. Pointing out that the law forbids sexual activity below a certain age, they are worried about anything that might – by stimulating children's natural curiosity – encourage sexual experimentation too early. Many also feel that the right place for sex education is the home, and that the right people to do it are parents themselves. Sex is an intimate subject, and one that is closely tied up with an adult's most deeply-felt moral and social values. The adults closest to the child are its parents, and passing values on is an important part of parenthood. So why should sex education be an exception?

Sometimes, people who support the principle of school sex education oppose the way it is done. Sexual activity, they say, is only morally acceptable when it takes place within the context of stable relationships (the reason being that these make the best background for bringing up children that result from the sex act). They condemn 'mechanical' sex education, which describes the physical aspects of sex but ignores the emotional, moral and social ones.

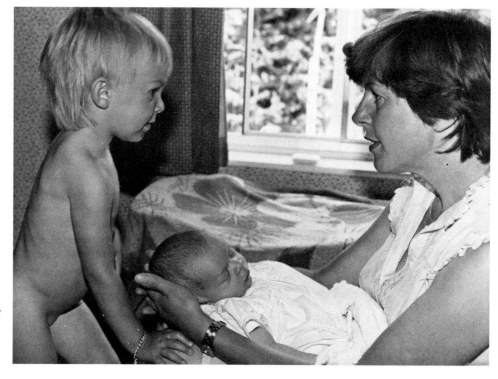

'The right place for sex education is the home.' Loving and intimate, a setting like this one is ideal for helping children to understand the facts of their own bodies. But what happens in families where love and intimacy are lacking?

the family?

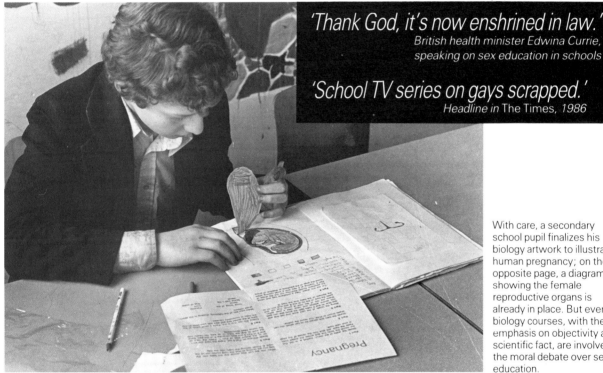

'Thank God, it's now enshrined in law.'
British health minister Edwina Currie,
speaking on sex education in schools

'School TV series on gays scrapped.'
Headline in The Times, 1986

With care, a secondary school pupil finalizes his biology artwork to illustrate human pregnancy; on the opposite page, a diagram showing the female reproductive organs is already in place. But even biology courses, with their emphasis on objectivity and scientific fact, are involved in the moral debate over sex education.

Totally unacceptable? Further problems arise when a sex education programme touches on an aspect of sexual activity that parents find unacceptable. Roman Catholics, for example, are deeply opposed to abortion and most forms of birth control. Many people of all beliefs do not approve of homosexuality. Should their children have to absorb views and beliefs which they themselves totally reject?

Can you count on them? It is often argued that leaving sex education to parents would be ideal ... if parents could be counted on to do it. As things are, many are too embarrassed to talk about the subject with their children (boys in particular lose out here), while some are too ignorant. In addition, countless families exist where little talking takes place at all. Does this mean that many children should have to be condemned to gleaning the 'facts of life' from school gossip or what they see in the media?

Sex education, its supporters point out, is not sex instruction. A properly planned sex education programme will introduce pupils to all aspects of a subject that's crucially important to them, and it will do so in a way that's appropriate to their level. What they learn will consist of accurate facts, rather than playground lore or misunderstood news stories. Furthermore, the people giving the lessons are trained to teach; since parents trust them with subjects like religious education, why can't teachers be trusted with sex education as well?

Mercy killing –

W as King George V murdered? This startling question was put before the world's historians in late 1986, when a writer disclosed the notes made by the British king's doctor as he attended his critically ill patient in the mid-1930s.

'Old people who feel that they're a burden to others, rightly or wrongly, might feel they would be "better away" for the sake of the younger generation . . . That would be an intolerable burden for an awful lot of old people.'

Dr Colin Currie, geriatrician

The doctor, Lord Dawson, had been told by the king's wife and eldest son that they did not want George's life prolonged if he was near the point of death. After the king had slid into a coma, Dawson decided that the moment had come; between eleven and midnight on the evening of 20 January, 1936, he ended the king's life with an injection of cocaine and morphia. The time was important: according to his own record, Dawson chose it so that news of the king's death could be first reported in the morning papers, rather than the 'less appropriate' evening ones.

George V may have been the most august person to have met his end this century through 'mercy killing' or euthanasia. But, although euthanasia is counted by the law as murder, he was certainly not the only one. People whose deaths have also been hastened for humane reasons include the incurably ill and unconscious, the senile, the grossly deformed new-born, and others who are not in a position to decide for themselves whether they want to live or not. Usually, the 'murderer' is a member of one of the medical professions.

Did Dawson and all his colleagues do right?

Right Fighting for the right to die: an elderly lady puts the case for publishing a controversial booklet on 'self-deliverance' at a meeting of Exit, now Britain's Voluntary Euthanasia Society. Behind her, the society's banner sums up an aspiration of millions, old and young.

or playing God?

A question of dignity? Now that people expect to live to fairly advanced ages, many actively dread the prospect of finally sinking into a vegetable existence: out of pain, perhaps, but unable to care for themselves, and unable to organize their own suicide. The knowledge that someone might then intervene to bring them to a peaceful and dignified end would, they feel, be immensely reassuring.

For many others, it is the prospect of severe illness and its treatment that inspires

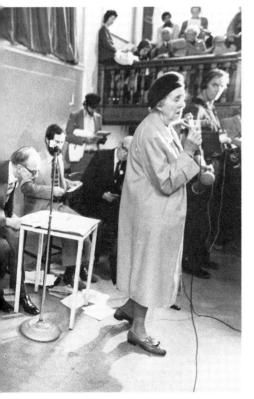

dread. Medical science can now do much to keep people alive who, even recently, would have died. However, a severely ill patient might welcome the chance to be allowed to die, rather than continuing to receive treatment that was painful or distressing.

Babies who are born with very severe deficiencies present the same dilemma. If they are kept alive, would their lives be happy? People often find it hard to blame a doctor or nurse who allow children like this to die.

Who can tell? Those who oppose euthanasia stress that it is murder, even if it is done for humane reasons. Human life is sacred, and no one has the right to play God by deciding when life should cease.

No one, too, can tell when surer or less painful treatments for diseases may be found – and no one can tell, either, whether a severely disabled child may not win through to a rewarding life.

Many people also feel that appalling abuses would follow if this form of murder were legalized. Would old people, for instance, be pressured by mercenary relatives to opt for euthanasia? In addition, the example of the Nazis' programmes of mass murder on 'eugenic' grounds is still clearly remembered.

'We always kept a bucket of water in the corner for cases like that.'
Former country midwife, remembering the birth of unviable children

Suicide: the

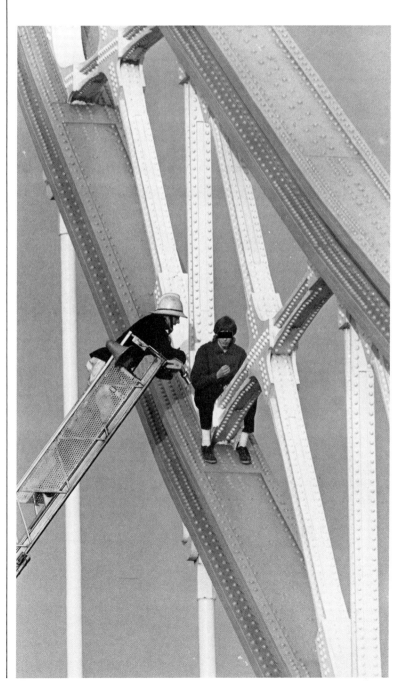

T

he final act that anyone can do with their own body is to destroy it. Depending on where – and when – you live, suicide is viewed with violently contrasting feelings. It has often been regarded as both a sin and a crime. It has also been seen as the peak of honourable self-sacrifice. More prosaically, many view it as the ultimate way to escape from intolerable difficulties.

A supreme gift destroyed? If you believe human life is the supreme gift of God, then destroying it wilfully is one of the worst things you can do. However desperate you are, 'playing God' with your own life is just as bad as playing it with other people's. You have no means of knowing what God's purpose is for you; whatever it is, however, you will frustrate it if you kill yourself.

Even people who are not religious are appalled by the finality of suicide. Once a person is dead, there is nothing at all that can be done to help them. If only they had been able to bear the pain of their illness, the humiliation of their mistakes, or the grief of a loved one's departure, things might have got better in future. Medicine, for example, is making continual progress. Now, however, it is too late.

Many think that killing oneself is the ultimate in cowardice. Putting this another way, suicide is the ultimate in refusing to take responsibility for oneself as a human being. Mistakes, though painful at the time, can be of advantage to those who make them, since they are part of the learning process. There is nothing to be gained by rejecting the new insights that they bring.

In addition, suicide is atrociously hard on the dead person's family and friends. The guilt they feel may well be out of all proportion to their responsibility for the suicide's death. Because of this, threats to commit suicide are a particularly un-pleasant form of blackmail.

ultimate way out?

A cry for help? It is commonplace to call attempted suicide a 'cry for help'. But hospitals, for example, are notorious for giving failed suicides short shrift. At a time when someone is feeling desperately unhappy (and also very ill), hospital staff are often brusque to the point of brutality. Such treatment is yet one more denial of help to a person who obviously needs it – and has failed to find it elsewhere. But which is better: to struggle on uncomplainingly against one's difficulties, or to express one's grief and rage in a way that must be heard?

The code of the samurai? In some cultures, suicide is not seen as wrong, but the reverse. The most famous example is probably the Japanese one. Under the samurai code of feudal Japan, it was the peak of honour to kill oneself rather than submit to humiliation or defeat.

The tradition of choosing suicide rather than dishonour has persisted into modern times: many Japanese soldiers killed themselves after World War Two rather than surrender to the Allies.

Opposite Threatening to jump? Amongst the dizzying girders of London's Tower Bridge, a fireman talks to a young man who took up station there on Christmas Eve, 1985. Eventually, both descended safely.

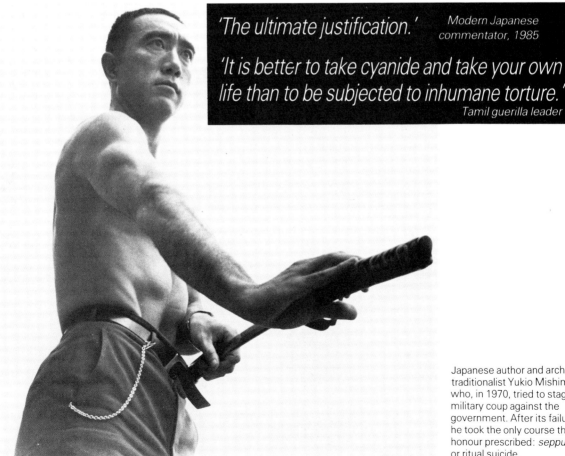

'The ultimate justification.' *Modern Japanese commentator, 1985*

'It is better to take cyanide and take your own life than to be subjected to inhumane torture.' *Tamil guerilla leader*

Japanese author and arch-traditionalist Yukio Mishima who, in 1970, tried to stage a military coup against the government. After its failure, he took the only course that honour prescribed: *seppuku*, or ritual suicide.

For their own good?

All societies make arrangements of some sort to care for people who, in ordinary life, cannot care for themselves: the old, the mentally ill or disabled, the physically handicapped. Much of the special care these people receive is focused on protecting them against physical danger.

> 'Some guests are in straitjackets or armmuffs, one guest is strapped to his bed. Technically they can leave if they apply in writing, but some have no powers of volition, some can't write, and some haven't got their arms free.'
> *Kathleen Jones and Alison Poletti, describing an Italian mental hospital in* New Society

However, the protective measures are often highly restrictive, and it is often argued that the carers go too far.

Where another category of helpless people – prisoners – are concerned, a more sinister situation exists. It is widely felt that, to keep them quiet and prevent trouble to others, prisoners are given tranquillizers and other drugs that they do not need.

How far should any carer interfere with the autonomy and physical freedom of cared-for individuals 'for their own good'?

Treated like children? Old age pensioners living in homes for the elderly can often feel they are treated like children. They are 'processed': got up, fed, sat in chairs before the television, medicated, fed again, finally hustled off to bed at a time more suited to a ten-year-old than a (frequently wakeful)

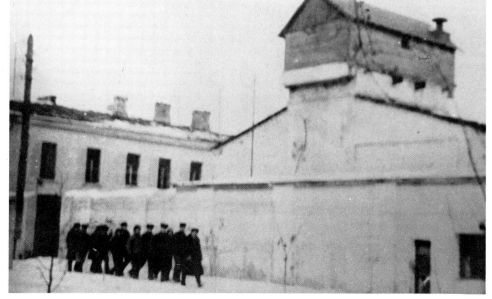

Russians who hold dissenting views risk being declared criminally insane, and sentenced to detention and 'treatment' in psychiatric hospitals like the one shown here. (The photograph was taken secretly.) 'If you talk too much,' comments one eye-witness, 'you get an injection of sulphazin, which sends your temperature up to 40°C and you are immobilised.'

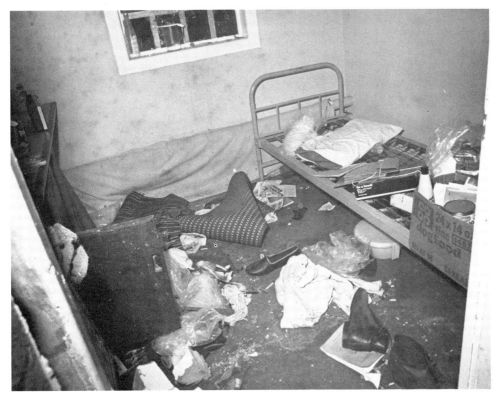

The aftermath of the 1978 riot at Gartree prison, Leicester. Inmates of Gartree feared that drugs were being used on a prisoner who had been taken to the jail's hospital. They asked to see him; when permission was refused, the riot erupted.

geriatric. In the interests of convenience and overall efficiency, staff may pay little real attention to inmates' individual needs and tastes. Complaints are brushed aside, nonconformist behaviour scolded out of existence. As a result, the residents are reduced to the state of feeding, sleeping vegetables, robbed of all responsibility for their actions and the dignity this confers.

If an over-practical approach can denude the helpless of dignity, so can an over-protective one. This often shows itself particularly strongly when a disabled person, for instance, wishes to form a sexual relationship or get married. Many people would say it was monstrous that someone should be discouraged from emotional independence just because they were blind or haemophiliac – or mentally handicapped.

If guiding a blind person away from marriage is an infringement of personal liberty, abusing the total powerlessness of prisoners is considerably worse. In British prisons, tranquillizers are called the 'liquid cosh', and many prisoners have claimed that they are over-used for just this reason. The opposite – forestalling criticism by under-prescribing drugs – is arguably almost as bad: in both cases, it is the demands of the institution that is controlling the authorities' actions, not those of the patient's condition.

The good of the community? Anyone who runs an institution would say that compromises have to be reached between the good of the individual and the good of the whole community. The zombie-like OAP is at least warm, well-fed, comfortable and safe from dangers like falling downstairs in his or her own home. The drugged prisoner is at least not beating up other prisoners or members of staff. Both are also cheaper to care for in staff terms than their freely active counterparts (all institutions have budgets).

It can also be pointed out that anyone counselling a disabled couple against potential marriage and parenthood would only have the couple's best interests at heart – and that of the children they might have.

'Three Appeal Court judges in London yesterday ordered that a 17 year old girl, with a mental age of about 5, should be sterilized for her own good.'

The Independent, *17 March, 1987*

Whose

Opposite Melissa Stern, the American child at the centre of the world-famous 'Baby M' case, with her father. The baby's biological mother, who had signed a surrogacy agreement with the Sterns, refused to give Baby M over to them. In early 1987, a judge ruled that the Sterns would offer the best home to the baby and should have her. But in a similar case in Britain, the judgement went the other way.

F or centuries, doctors have been aware of the possibilities of using 'borrowed' organs (real or artificial) in treatment. Until recently, they lacked the knowledge and technology to make this work. Now they have both, and the sophistication of their techniques is growing year by year.

Public acceptance of their achievements, however, has not always kept pace with the achievements themselves. Many legal and ethical problems have yet to be solved, some of them extremely complex. The most complex of all are probably those surrounding the most fundamental of all human relationships: the tie between a child and its parents.

New hope? Under normal circumstances, parenthood starts when an egg is fertilized inside the mother's body by the father's sperm. As livestock breeders have known for many years, sperm can be stored outside the male body and still maintain their fertility. When needed, they can be used to fertilize the mother artificially (AID – artificial insemination by donor). Now the

'The funny thing is that people keep saying how like my husband they look.'
Mother of three children conceived by AID

technology also exists for IVF – in vitro fertilization, or the fertilization of the egg by the father's sperm outside the mother's body. Once fertilized, the 'test-tube baby' is implanted in the mother's womb and develops normally.

AID and IVF have brought new hope to many married couples who would have otherwise remained infertile. AID – with sperm from a different donor – can be used where the husband is sterile; IVF when ordinary conception is very difficult. Both have attracted criticism; the child of an AID conception, for instance, is technically illegitimate, while IVF arouses in many the instinctive feeling that it 'isn't natural'. However, this feeling is mild compared to those aroused by another way of becoming a parent altogether: surrogacy.

A denial of human dignity? A 'surrogate mother' undertakes to carry and bear a baby for someone else: typically, for a man and a woman who are desperate to have a child of their own, but cannot have one together. For the service, she is paid a fee.

In the United States, surrogacy is legal, although it is being challenged in the courts. In some other countries, the payment of fees is banned, and the whole principle of surrogacy could be banned as well. One objection is that it is fundamentally unworkable. Whatever the surrogate mother may undertake before becoming pregnant, her feelings could undergo a deep change during pregnancy and birth. Given the importance of early bonding, forcing her to give up her baby then would be grossly inhumane.

In America, opponents of surrogacy contracts have said that these are simply baby-selling in another form. Everywhere, indeed, many people would agree that to make a profit out of breeding human beings is a fundamental denial of human rights and dignity.

womb?

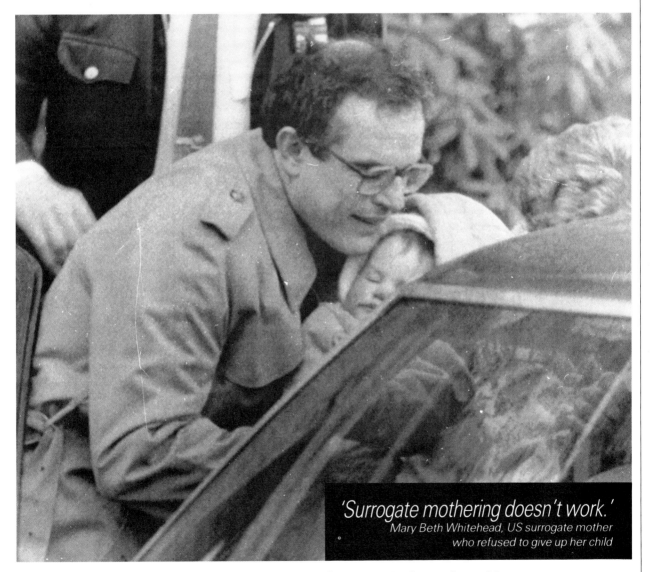

'Surrogate mothering doesn't work.'
*Mary Beth Whitehead, US surrogate mother
who refused to give up her child*

Her own womb? It can be argued that the surrogate mother's womb is her own, to do as she wishes with. If she wishes to have a baby, and then hand it over to someone else, what is wrong with that? Infertility is the source of much human misery. If having a baby for an infertile couple would end their distress, does this gain not outweigh other considerations? Just because a solution is new does not mean that it is unacceptable.

Parts to

igh on television's list of great fiction heroes is a figure known to young viewers across the world as the Six Million Dollar Man: a hideously injured astronaut who – thanks to spare-part surgery – was reconstructed as a super-human. Television's Bionic Man is still technically in the future; however, the technology does exist to give new hip joints to crippled people, new eyes to the blind, and new hearts and lungs to the dying. The hip joints are artificially made but, as yet, the best substitutes for most human organs are other human organs.

Organ transplants are much more common than they were, but both surgeons

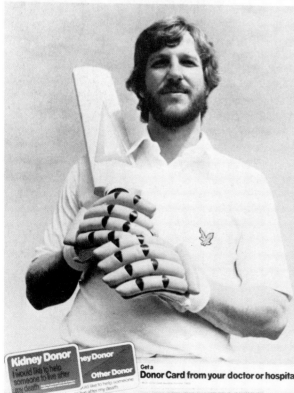

Ian Botham says 'I would like to help someone to live after my death.'

Kidney Donor
I would like to help someone to live after my death
Other Donor

Get a **Donor Card** from your doctor or hospital

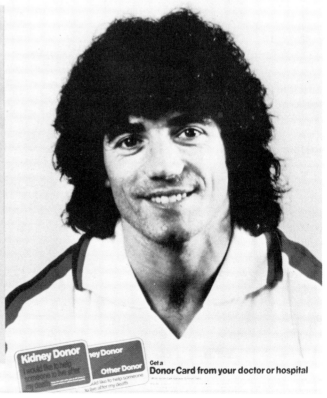

Kevin Keegan says 'I would like to help someone to live after my death.'

Kidney Donor
I would like to help someone to live after my death
Other Donor

Get a **Donor Card** from your doctor or hospital

spare?

and patients are still bedevilled by spare part shortages.

The life-saver? Most people readily accept that organ transfer is an essential part of modern medicine. It not only saves lives, it also – as all kidney transplant patients can vouch – radically transforms the quality of life. (Anyone who knows a kidney disease patient on dialysis also knows how restricted a life the patient lives, tied as he or she is to the life-saving sessions on the machine.)

Organ transfer can be particularly rewarding in the case of the very young, who can have a whole future assured to them by the surgeon's skill. Here, the donors naturally have to be young as well. Although their death is heart-breaking to their parents, these have often found comfort in the fact that some good is coming out of their child's death.

Reassured? In the early days of transplants, many people feared that doctors eager for this or that organ would take them from a donor's body while the donor was still alive. Much work, however, has now been done on defining death and the current definition – brain death – has been proved infallible to most people's satisfaction. Thus reassured, many people are prepared to donate some of their organs to medicine, as is proved by the speed with which volunteer 'organ donor' cards disappear from the pick-up points where they are displayed in shops and elsewhere.

Too distraught? However – and even despite the dead person's wishes – many people are too distraught on the death of a

loved one to think of authorizing an organ donation. Many, too, would feel distressed at the best of times at the idea of having the body of their child or spouse 'cut about'. A few Christians, meanwhile, believe that the body literally rises from the dead in the state in which it was buried, and reject the idea of organ donation on those grounds. For all these reasons, doctors and nurses are often very reluctant to bring up the question of organ donation with grieving relatives – even though they well know how urgent the need is.

Opposite The plastic message of hope: in this 1980 campaign to encourage organ donation, posters feature leading sportsmen Ian Botham and Kevin Keegan. Like them, most people would like to help someone to live after their deaths; so why do patients often have to wait so long for an organ transfer operation?

> *'We are identifying foetuses so fatally damaged that survival outside the womb is impossible. The ability to transplant foetal organs may now give us the chance to recognize the contribution of this doomed foetus to mankind.'*
> Dr Michael Harrison, University of California, 1986

> *'If the baby was not officially dead then it was alive and removing his heart is murder.'*
> John Scarisbrick, chairman of the anti-abortion organization Life

However, the question that continues to dominate people's concern remains the definition of death. In both the USA and Britain, this has recently been given new impetus by the use for transplant of organs from babies born without brains. Without a brain, how can death be measured?

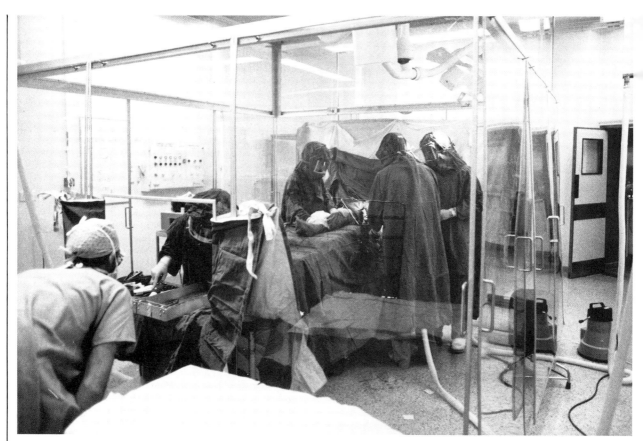

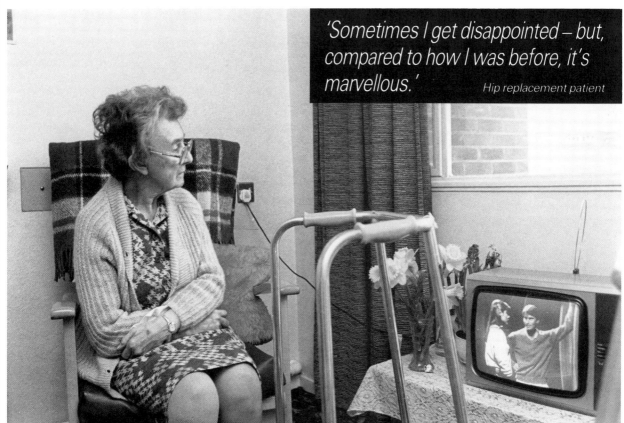

'Sometimes I get disappointed – but, compared to how I was before, it's marvellous.'

Hip replacement patient

Out of joint?

Another controversy over spare-part surgery focuses, not on where the parts come from, but on the cost of giving them to their new owners. Compared to many other medical achievements, this can be high, even in the case of comparatively less complex operations such as hip replacements. The cost factor is often the reason why long queues exist for spare-part surgery; how far is this justified?

Goodbye to pain? Most people today know at least one person whose life has been transformed by the insertion of a plastic kneecap or titanium hip joint. Patients like these can walk, bicycle, sleep well at night, go to work, and throw their pain-killers away. Until relatively recently, however, all these things would have been impossible for them. Without spare-part surgery, they would have led lives filled with severe pain. Walking, in particular, would have been a misery, even with a stick, and their forced immobility caused many extra problems. The quality of their whole life was affected by their disability.

A hip replacement, therefore, not only frees its recipient from misery. It also restores him or her to life that's worth living, just as surely as a heart transplant restores patients to life itself. In addition, it restores to society a valuable – because productive – member. Many people would say that, compared to arguments like these, the cost factor should not be allowed to carry disproportionate weight; what counts most is the physical and social welfare of the patient. It's also pointed out that the cost of any former breakthrough in medicine comes down as techniques advance.

Balancing the books? Doctors and medical administrators both agree that their aim is to help patients. However, they have to work within the limits of the possible, and these limits always include the financial ones. Patients who need the installation of a 'spare part', whether artificial or of human origin, form only a proportion of all the patients a doctor or a hospital has to deal with; they also form only a proportion of all the people in a community who fall ill. Both society and individual hospitals have a duty to balance their budgets, and the doctors have no option but to work within these.

> ## 'Cash shortage stops hip operations.'
> *Headline in* The Times, *1987*

Recently, people have begun to work out some exact ways of helping to make the books balance. For instance, only one person can benefit directly from a hip replacement operation. But, by spending the same sum of money on a 'risks of smoking' education programme, a doctor could bring a similar amount of benefit to 120 people. If there is enough cash for both the operation and the programme, well and good. But, if money is tight, is it right to help a few people at the expense of the many?

Opposite (top) An immaculately clean environment is extra-crucial for hip replacements. Here, a patient has a new hip fitted in a 'room within a room'; the surgeons, equipped like divers, are being fed air from outside. But special hygiene precautions like these only push the cost of a hip replacement up still further.

Opposite (bottom) A huge gulf separates the active youngsters on the screen and the elderly lady watching them. For the nearly immobile, a walking-frame is both a cage and the key to (very limited) freedom; how much would alternatives cost?

The blood

The idea of blood transplants – or transfusions – goes back a long way. People were giving successful blood transfusions to animals in the seventeenth century; the first successful one with humans took place in 1829, and the later discovery of blood groups ensured that thousands of lives could be saved by transfusions during the First World War.

Today, medicine would be unthinkably handicapped if it could not rely on blood donor programmes and blood banks. And – in the developed world at least – most people have come to take blood transfusions and their life-saving role for granted. However, this feeling is not shared by everyone. Why?

Forbidden in the Bible? Some religious sects believe that, even though blood transfusions may save life, they are forbidden in the Bible. They therefore reject anything involving the transfer of other people's blood to their own bodies.

People who do not share these beliefs usually regard them with incomprehension and dismay. They accept that, in a free society, everyone should be able to follow their own religious beliefs. But they strongly question whether this should extend to withholding life-saving treatment from individuals who need it.

To give – or to sell? With the development of artificial blood substitute for transfusions, the problems over religious beliefs have been reduced. However, another controversy over blood transfusion now exists that could get increasingly fiercer. It concerns, not those who receive other people's blood, but those who give it. In some countries – Britain is an example – all blood is given free. Donors get no reward other than the feeling that they have done something to help other people. Elsewhere, giving blood to a blood bank is a commercial enterprise.

In the US, for instance, many suppliers get paid for their donation, while others do it to work off a 'blood debt': the obligation run up by a relative who has already had a transfusion. The rules the Americans build into their system have been particularly effective in producing plasma for blood products such as Factor VIII: the substance used by haemophiliacs to help their blood clot.

Opponents of 'blood for hire' point out, however, that paid donors have everything to gain and nothing to lose from concealing things that might make their blood unsuitable: a history of drug addiction, for

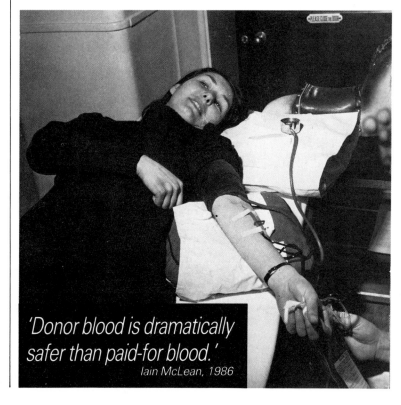

Opposite The average adult contains about eight pints – or five litres – of blood. Heavy blood loss, like that suffered by victims of many road accidents, could prove fatal if blood banks and their stored contents did not exist, ready for use in just such emergencies.

The 'gift relationship' in action, here linking London with Vietnam. The young donor – a French *au pair* girl – is giving blood to help casualties on both sides of the Vietnam War of the 1960s and 1970s.

'Donor blood is dramatically safer than paid-for blood.'
Iain McLean, 1986

# of others?

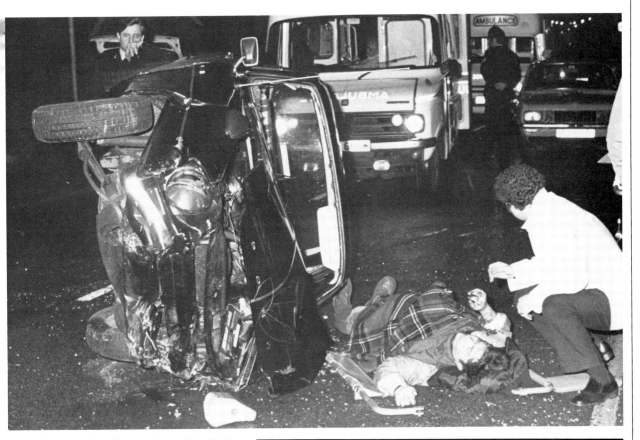

example, or the disease hepatitis B. In addition, drug addicts or alcoholics might be more attracted than most people to making quick and easy money by selling their blood.

Arguments like these have been running for many years, but they have been given new importance by the spread of AIDS. Many now fear that a paid donor service could bring grave risk to people who have to use blood products like Factor VIII. Already Americans who have had multiple blood transfusions since the mid-1970's, are facing the prospect of compulsory AIDS tests.

'Their sorrows shall be multiplied that hasten after another god: their drink offerings of blood will I not offer, nor take up their names into my lips.'

King David, Psalm 16:4 – the text that Jehovah's Witnesses take as their justification for rejecting blood transfusions

Well, whose illness is it?

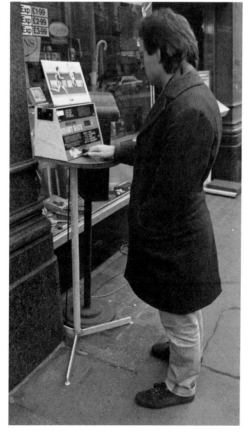

Opposite A herbalist at work. Herbalism is a branch of medicine that is often labelled 'alternative' or complementary; other examples include acupuncture and osteopathy. The aim of alternative medicine is to treat the whole person, not just the disease. Many Western people are turning to it because they are dissatisfied with 'mainstream' medical practice.

Taking charge of one's own health – with a little help from modern technology. For a non-medic, taking one's own pulse is notoriously difficult. But a public 'Check your heart rate' machine gives the layman easy access to this vital bit of information.

We are never so aware of our bodies as when there is something wrong with them. Yet that is also the time when we have least control over them. With our willing – and usually eager – consent, they have to be handed over to those who are legally qualified to treat them, and to their vast army of helpers.

We are naturally grateful to anyone who rescues us from pain, and delighted if we can be restored to full health. Many of us, too, have nothing but praise for the people who do it. Equally, however, many of us have dismal tales to tell of our treatment at the hands of doctors, receptionists, nurses and other medical staff. Patients are treated brusquely, told they're 'imagining things', or have their requests ignored. Anxious relatives are fobbed off. Children are frightened out of their wits by horrors that no one has time to explain.

Based on a myth? Stirred by miseries like these, more and more people are now beginning to challenge the people who inflict them. Many patients no longer feel it is right that the medical professions should exercise such unquestioned power. The old motto of 'doctor knows best' is now being replaced with a new one: 'I want to take charge of my own illness'.

For a start, it can be argued that a doctor's reputation of omnipotence – along with the docile respect it commands – is based on a myth. Very often, the patient is not 'cured' by the doctor, but by his or her own natural powers of recuperation. The doctor merely manages these and, in the view of many, often uses methods that are unnecessarily drastic to do it.

Again, the person who is having the illness is the patient, not the doctor. The doctor has been asked to advise the patient on what to do – but that is all. He or she has not been invited to make a take-over bid for the patient's body and mind.

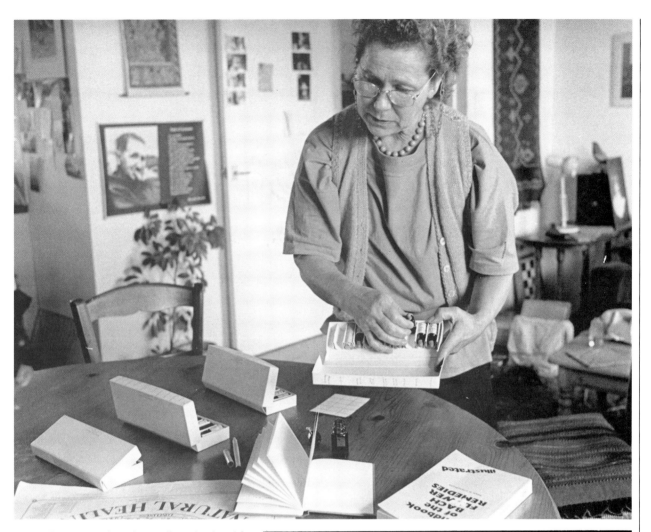

The business of getting well again should, people now feel, involve an equal partnership between doctor and patient. And, since patients have to live with the results of what the doctor suggests, they should certainly have all the facts and choices carefully explained to them.

'The good of my patients?' All doctors, however they are perceived by their patients, are working with one aim in view: the patient's own benefit. The famous Hippocratic Oath – allegedly composed by the father of western medicine over two thousand years ago – sums up their intentions: 'I will prescribe regimen for the good of my patients according to my ability and my judgement and never do harm to anyone.' Other medical and paramedical staff would own to similar goals.

With the best of intentions, however, the professions involved often find it difficult to communicate with patients in addition to treating them. There is often no time. Or

> *'I think children should be told everything doctors tell parents, however complicated. We are the ones going through it.'*
> Hospital patient, aged 13

> *'She understands what I say, listens to what I say, does what I say, believes what I say.'*
> US doctor describing the perfect patient

the patient may be too difficult to approach, too frightened, too young, too old, or too under-educated or uninterested to grasp difficult concepts and terms. Or everyone may be just too tired to do more than their basic job. And this, doctors point out, is curing people. While they acknowledge a patient might appreciate a more human approach, they are not in business to be public relations experts.

Shouldn't

In many countries, patients have two sorts of control over their own illness. They not only have the right to accept treatment or reject it; they also have the right to know exactly what they are being treated for. In Sweden, Australia and the USA, for example, people are by law entitled to see the records that doctors hold on them, and to read what the doctors have said. Recent European legislation on computer data is leading to the same right being established for British patients. However, the issue has been hotly fought over, with British doctors defending their established practice of keeping their notes on patients to themselves.

Distressed to no purpose? The doctors rest their case on their view of what is best for the patient. If, for example, the file of notes on a patient shows that cancer has been diagnosed, this knowledge may distress the patient unbearably. Worse, the patient may be distressed to no purpose, since the diagnosis might be wrong.

Again, doctors often make personal comments on patients – 'Nervous' or 'Uncooperative', for example – which could be of use to anyone else treating them. Until recently, these remarks have been jotted down in the absolute certainty that the patient will never get to see them, and some are very blunt indeed. As a result, the doctors now feel at risk from being sued for libel.

They also point out that most laymen would be baffled by the contents of their personal files, since these are expressed in medical terms. Explaining them to someone who lacks medical training (and probably any scientific knowledge as well) would take up a great deal of time – time that could best be spent on treating patients rather than running information sessions for them.

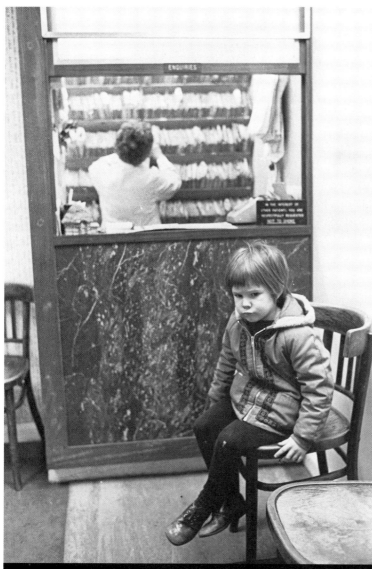

'When we deliberately conceal the truth from an adult we are in effect treating him as a child.'

Professor Christopher Dickinson, 1986

they tell us ?

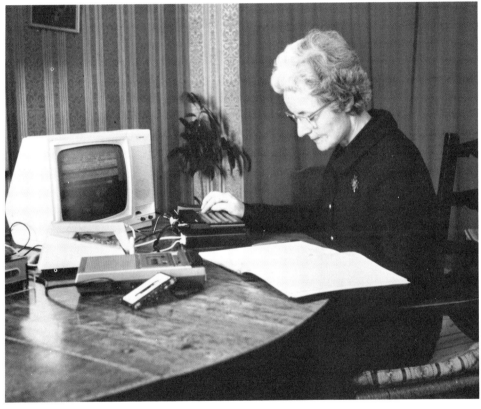

Opposite Shut out? This child would not expect to read the medical file that exists on her. But, in Britain, most adults now find it shocking that they, too, are debarred from seeing what the doctor has written about them. As things stood in early 1987, few patients had even held their medical records in their hands. How many, for example, know that the final space on a file like the ones shown here is headed 'Cause of death?'

The agent of change: the computer, here used by a nurse for entering details of her casework. Under European law, everyone has the right to examine computer data held on them. Some British patients are therefore gaining access to their own medical files – but most files are still the old-style, hand-written ones.

Professional arrogance? Some doctors, however, share the view taken by almost all patients. The body under discussion is the patient's, so he or she has a right to know about it. It is outrageous for any professionals, however well-intentioned, to hug to themselves the knowledge they come by about the patient's body. Their reluctance to share it with the body's owner is yet one more proof of the professional arrogance that many are felt to show.

Most people who fear they have a serious disease would wish the doctor to tell them what is really wrong with them. Worrying about what the doctor is concealing can in itself be bad for health. Furthermore, all patients would welcome the chance to correct any inaccuracies they spot on their records, and to put their own point of view when the doctor has labelled them unco-operative or worse.

Forcing doctors to explain what they are doing (and why) will improve medical care, because it will help reinforce the idea of the doctor-patient partnership that is now beginning to take root.

> *'The work involved in providing medical access whereby we have to write reports will be a bureaucratic nightmare.'*
> *Paddy Ross, British Medical Association*

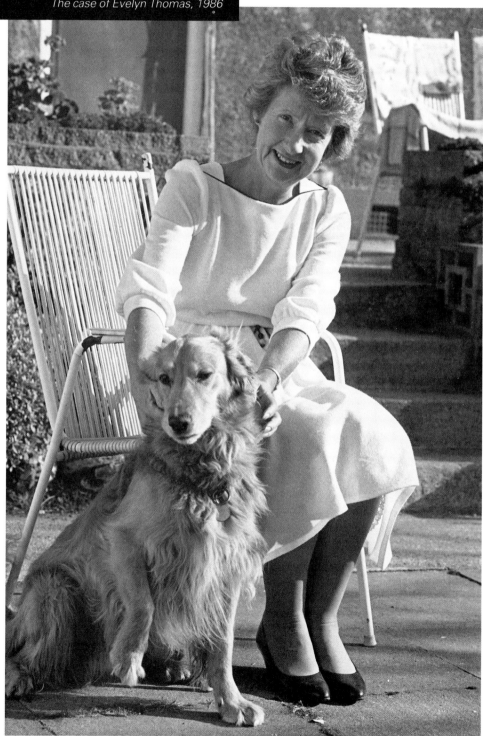

'Unknown to Mrs Thomas, and without her informed consent, she had been entered into the trial which meant that for a year the counsellor was not allowed to approach her.'

The case of Evelyn Thomas, 1986

Who wants to be a guinea pig?

However much doctors and patients may disagree over some aspects of caring for the human body, there are quite a few subjects on which they are united. One of the most important involves the safety of the treatment that doctors hand out and that patients undergo. No patient would wish to be exposed to a treatment that had not been thoroughly tested for safety, and no doctor would wish to prescribe one.

However, this raises a problem. There is a limit to the extent to which medical treatments for humans can be usefully tested on animals, always supposing that such tests are ethically acceptable in the first place. So they have to be tested on humans. Is it right to treat humans as guinea-pigs, even if (as is sometimes not the case) they are willing subjects?

Do they know what they're doing? Many people would say that testing on human volunteers is acceptable, as long as the volunteers fully understand what they are doing. They should be aware that a medical trial is a journey into the unknown. Do they know what is involved, and are they really prepared to take any risks that come?

> 'Aids tests without consent urged.' *Headline in* The Independent, *February 1987*

Indeed, do they know what the risks are, or what compensation (if any) they would get if they are harmed?

It can be argued that the testers enter a murkier field in cases where the volunteers' partial ignorance is essential to the test. This happens very frequently. It is pointless, for example, to test the performance of a certain drug unless this performance is compared with something else: perhaps the performance of another drug, or perhaps the effects of receiving no treatment whatsoever.

However, people have strong powers of 'thinking' their bodies into reacting as their minds would expect. For this reason, volunteers are not told whether they are taking the new drug, an established one, or a harmless substitute called a 'placebo'. Although an accepted part of all testing, does this forced ignorance run counter to the right of individuals to control what happens to their bodies?

Cases where subjects do not know they are being involved in a test present an even greyer area still. It does happen – and many people would say that, however good the motives of the testers, it represents a totally unacceptable infringement of individual liberties.

Who suffers most? The fact remains that no one would wish to accept a medical (or any other) treatment that had not been thoroughly tested for possible bad effects. Which involves the most suffering: possible damage to the bodies or feelings of a few individuals (most of whom are volunteers anyway) or similar damage to hundreds of thousands, who in the matter of falling ill had no choice?

In the end, it comes down to the question of the greatest good of the greatest number.

Opposite Breast cancer patient and unwitting 'guinea pig' Evelyn Thomas, whose story appeared in *The Independent*. After she had had a mastectomy, Mrs Thomas hoped to receive the help of a trained nurse counsellor who never came. Mrs Thomas discovered later that a random trial was being held at the hospital on the benefits of counselling. Without knowing about it, she had been entered in the trial; as a result, a counsellor was not allowed near her for a year.

A judgement on the world?

Opposite Fighting for our lives: New York gays band together in support of AIDS victims. One positive result of the AIDS epidemic is the growth of caring networks and – amongst the wider public – compassion for those who have the disease.

Right Although few women in Britain have so far contracted AIDS, almost all are now aware that they are at the mercy of their sexual partners in this respect. Will the threat of AIDS drive women back into the restricted sexual life that society forced on them for centuries, and from which they have only just escaped? And how should a woman feel if she is given AIDS by her husband?

Twenty years after the 'liberal revolution' of the 1960s, a completely new factor hit the world's health programmes, legal systems and codes of morality: AIDS (Acquired Immune Deficiency Syndrome). By the end of 1986, almost 5,000 people had died of it in New York City alone – and one person in every 250 was estimated to carry the disease.

In Europe, the figures were much lower. In France, over 400 people had died; in West Germany, over 300; in Britain, just under 300. However, out of a British population of 56 million, a possible 40,000 were believed to carry the disease, and therefore to be in a position to give it to others. And, in spite of the efforts of the world's medical community, there was still no cure.

Who's at risk? From the time the disease first became known in the western world, AIDS was linked in people's minds with sexual behaviour and, in particular, with homosexuality. Statistics show that, in developed countries, homosexual men run a much heavier risk of contracting the disease than heterosexual ones. So do people who inject themselves with drugs;

so do those who have had sexual intercourse with people living in Central Africa, where the disease is common and (although this is not certain) where it probably started. Sufferers from haemophilia are also threatened, since they rely for treatment on blood products that may have come from donors infected with AIDS.

The AIDS virus, which is carried in blood, semen and vaginal fluid, is transmitted through sexual contact, so the sexual partners of everyone in the 'at risk' categories themselves run the risk of catching the disease. And, if they themselves have other

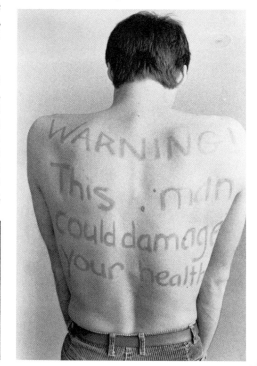

'Everyone detected with AIDS should be tattooed in the upper forearm, to protect common needle users, and in the buttocks to prevent the victimisation of other homosexuals.' *William Buckley*, New York Times *columnist*

sexual partners, they can also pass it on.

The new lepers? Because of the apparent speed and ease with which the disease can be spread, those who suffer from it have become the modern equivalent of lepers. AIDS is feared even more than other deadly diseases, such as cancer and rabies. In their hearts, many people view it as an expression of the wrath of God: a punishment for breaking sexual taboos that, until the 1960s, were sacred. The fact that the AIDS virus can be found in other body fluids, such as saliva, has only added to the general panic. In Britain the panic was given an extra twist by the discovery that one sufferer caught it from a skin graft.

The fear of AIDS is so great that people have begun to react very strongly to anything they see as a threat. In the USA, Californians were asked to ban all carriers of the AIDS virus from jobs that brought them into contact with other people; New Yorkers tried to get two schools to cross AIDS-infected children off their rolls. Both attempts failed; in Britain, however, parents did temporarily keep their children away from a school with an AIDS-infected pupil. British TV technicians refused to work inside the premises of an organization founded to help AIDS victims. And insurance companies are beginning to refuse cover to people who they think may be homosexual.

Given that there is no cure, these fears are understandable. But – especially in the case of the children involved – is it possible to justify their effects on those who carry the AIDS virus?

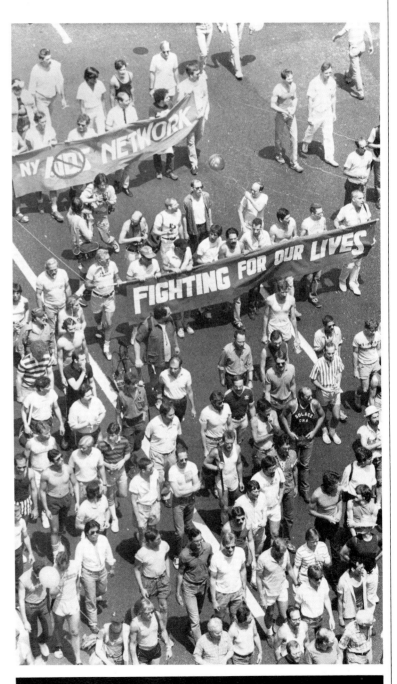

'I thought they were going to come and daub our house with a red cross.'
Mother of (school-age) AIDS virus carrier

A new morality?

Because of the way AIDS is transmitted, it is indissolubly linked in people's minds with questions of morality – and, because people are frightened, their feelings on the subject are very strong. They are so strong, in fact, that the western world's ideas of acceptable sexual behaviour seem to be changing almost overnight. We could be witnessing a second moral revolution, as far-reaching in its effects as its 1960s predecessor. But what does this new 'morality' consist of? How far does it balance the legitimate needs of society with those of the individual? Will the end result be for our benefit, or the reverse?

Does it serve them right? Amongst people with conventional views on sexual morality, attitudes to AIDS sufferers are currently ranging from deep distress and compassion to a blunt 'Serves you right'. No one, whatever their views, withholds sympathy from the so-called 'innocent' victims of the dis-

Opposite 'What you ought to know about AIDS' a booklet that was distributed free to all West German homes in 1985. In the absence of a cure, the only hope of controlling the disease lies in conquering ignorance about it.

Dead of the plague: man, horse, hound, and the birds of the air. In this engraving by the medieval artist Hans Brueghel, only the doctor and the sorrowing woman have not yet been affected. The most infamous of the great historical plague epidemics was the Black Death, which killed a third of the people in the world. The terror it caused is today closely paralleled by public panic over AIDS – almost as mysterious to us in its workings, and (so far) equally incurable.

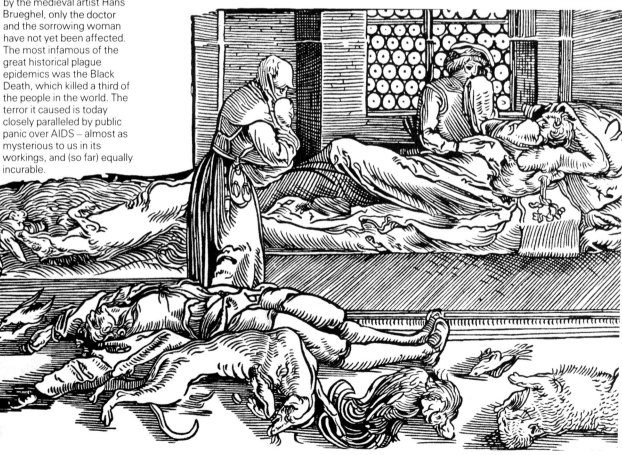

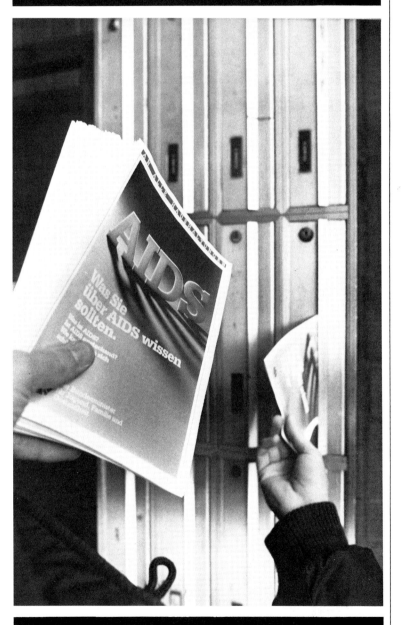

ease: the haemophilia sufferers treated with tainted Factor VIII, the babies infected with AIDS in the womb, and others. Right across the board, the arguments in favour of sexual restraint and responsibility are now over-whelming.

Return to repression? For all those, how-ever, who welcomed the liberalizing effects of the first moral revolution, the repressive results of the second are dismaying. In a matter of months, AIDS has: re-charged the sexual act with fear and guilt; re-smirched homosexuals with a stigma as bad as the one they have now escaped; robbed women of their hard-won control over the effects of sex on their own bodies; and given powerful ammunition to those who believe that sex-ual freedom is intrinsically wrong.

Just skin deep? In the face of the clinical evidence, it is now impossible to believe in the '60s ideal of sex with no tomorrows and no regrets. Promiscuity is hazardous, both to oneself and one's partners. 'Safe sex' is not as safe as all that, and real safety lies only in complete abstinence or fidelity to one sexual partner. For once, self-interest and the demands of society coincide.

It can be asked, however, how far the discovery of a cure would alter attitudes. Freed from fear, would the new morality still hold its supporters? Or would it prove to be skin deep? Is chastity intrinsically right, or merely an appropriate reaction in a situation that threatens our lives?

In addition, it is already worth asking whether the public outcry on AIDS would have been so loud if the disease had, say, been transmitted by animal bites, like rabies. Are we victims of our own fears, as well as of the disease? And which, in the end, will be the more powerful?

'Pairing and bonding are normally part of human nature, and promiscuity is contrary to it.' The Church of England Board for Social Responsibility

Reference

Glossary

Abortion – The ending of a pregnancy through the removal of the unborn child from the mother's womb. In the modern sense of the word, the removal is normally an artificially-induced process.

Addiction – Extremely severe dependence (physical, psychological or both) on a drug.

AID – Initials standing for 'artificial insemination by donor': the fertilization of a female by the artificial introduction into her body of male sperm. Often carried out in animal husbandry; more rarely with humans. Where the sperm introduced into a woman's body is that of her legal partner, the term is 'artificial insemination by husband' (AIH).

AIDS – Initials standing for 'acquired immune deficiency syndrome': a virus-caused disease that attacks the human body's own self-defence system. Carriers of the virus include semen and vaginal fluid; it can therefore be passed on through sexual activity with an infected person. At the time of writing – early 1987 – no cure was known.

Anaesthetics – Substances that give immunity to pain. A patient receiving a local anaesthetic will remain conscious, but will not feel pain caused by surgical treatment to a certain part of the body; a patient under general anaesthesia loses consciousness while treatment is carried out.

Anorexia nervosa – A psychological illness (usually affecting young women) that features extreme loss of appetite. Also known as the 'slimmers' disease'; has been known to cause death.

Birth control – Deliberate action taken by either partner in sexual intercourse to prevent a resulting pregnancy. Methods include the 'natural' (such as abstinence from intercourse, or the rhythm method), the mechanical (such as the condom), the oral ('the Pill') and the permanent (sterilization).

Black Death – The plague epidemic that devastated the world's populations and economies during the Middle Ages.

Blood transfusion – The introduction into a patient's body of blood from another human source. Usually, the blood introduced has been collected from its donor well before the transfusion and stored in a blood bank, although direct donor-to-patient transfusions are sometimes carried out.

Brain death – The point at which the brain of a dead person permanently ceases all activity; now the definition of the point of death in the case of potential organ donors. Even 'brain-dead' people, however, can have their circulation artificially maintained by medical equipment.

Bronchitis – Infection of the respiratory system. Chronic bronchitis, with breathlessness and a cough of long standing, is particularly associated with smoking.

Cancer (breast, cervix, lung and other) – Abnormality of cell growth resulting in malignant (spreading) tumours.

Cirrhosis – Disease of the liver often caused by alcohol addiction.

Cloning – A method of reproducing organisms by means that are a-sexual: not achieved through sexual intercourse. A plant grown from a cutting is a clone.

Condom – Rubber sheath placed over the penis during sexual intercourse. Its main use is as a contraceptive, but it also helps to act as a barrier against sexually-transmitted diseases such as AIDS.

Contraception – See 'Birth control'.

Contraceptive pill – Often simply known as 'the Pill', this method of birth control covers many varieties of hormone-based oral contraceptive.

Corporal punishment – The control of behaviour through the infliction of bodily pain; most typically, by beating.

Dialysis, renal – The mechanical removal from a kidney patient's bloodstream of waste products whose accumulation would otherwise prove fatal. Someone with kidney disease may have to spend 30 hours a week on a kidney machine.

Embryo – The unborn human, up to the age of two months from conception.

Eugenics – The application of selective breeding principles to human reproduction, with a view to improving or altering characteristics of the human race.

Euthanasia – Also called 'mercy killing', euthanasia involves the painless killing of individuals who are incurably ill or otherwise incapable of enjoying a rewarding life. Very frequently used with animals.

Factor VIII – Substance derived from blood that helps the blood of haemophiliacs to clot.

Foetus – The unborn human, from the age of two months after conception.

Genetic disorders – Abnormal conditions that have been handed on to the patient through his or her genetic make-up: the blend of genes inherited from earlier generations.

Geriatrics – The medical science of treating and caring for the elderly.

Haemophilia – A genetic disorder that prevents the patient's blood from clotting normally. It only affects men, but is passed to them by their mothers rather than their fathers.

Hepatitis B – Liver disease transmitted through infected blood.

Homosexuality – Sexual attraction felt for members of the same sex; often – but not invariably – linked with sexual intercourse with the object of attraction.

IVF – Initials standing for 'in vitro fertilization': the process whereby a woman's ovum is fertilized by a male sperm outside her body – typically, in a glass laboratory dish.

'Liberal Revolution' – The dramatic loosening-up of many aspects of morality – including sexual morality – that took place in the 1960s and 1970s. Also often called the 'permissive revolution' or the 'sexual revolution'.

Nicotine – Drug found in tobacco.

Obesity – The state of being too heavy for one's height, build and age; in general terms, the state of being too fat.

Ova – Egg cells carried in a female's body; when fertilized by a male sperm, an ovum (the singular form of 'ova') develops into an embryo.

Placebo – Non-active substance given to a patient, often with a view to 'deceiving' his or her body into feeling better.

Prohibition – When spelled with a capital 'P', refers to the nation-wide ban that the USA attempted to enforce between the wars on the sale and consumption of alcoholic drink.

Rabies – Disease of the nervous system; transmitted to humans through the bite of an infected ('rabid') animal.

Semen – The sperm-carrying fluid produced by the male during sexual intercourse.

'Spare-part surgery' – Surgical techniques that involve the replacement of a defective organ in the patient with a fully-functioning artificial one; in general speech, is often also used to cover surgical transplants of organs from human donors.

Spermatozoa – Often shortened to 'sperm'; the male fertilizing cells transmitted to the female during sexual intercourse. Fertilization takes place when a sperm unites with an ovum.

Sterilization – Surgical procedures that render males and females permanently incapable of becoming parents.

Suicide – The action whereby a person deliberately takes his or her own life.

Surrogate parenthood – Also called 'surrogacy', it involves an agreement between a fertile woman and a hitherto childless couple. The woman agrees to bear and give birth to a child that will be handed over to the couple to bring up as their own.

'Test-tube babies' – Children conceived through the IVF process.

Transplant surgery – The replacement of a patient's defective organ with a functioning organ taken from a human donor, living or dead.

Virus – Agents of infection; viruses are very much smaller than bacteria.

Further reading

BOOKS

Blood transfusions

The Gift Relationship by R. M. Titmuss (Allen & Unwin, 1970). The classic work on the (pre-AIDS) situation concerning supplies of blood for transfusion, it contrasts UK and US practice.

Contraception

The Bitter Pill by Dr Ellen Grant (Elm Tree Books, 1985/Corgi Pathway, 1986). The reasons why women give up using the contraceptive pill, based on 20 years' research on the pill's side-effects.

The Pill, a Handbook for Users by John Guillebaud (Oxford University Press, 1984). Both the pros and the cons, written by the medical director of the Margaret Pyke Centre, London, where different varieties of pill and other contraceptives are being tested at the time of writing.

Fertility and embryo research

Human Embryo Research: Yes or No by the CIBA Foundation (Tavistock Publications, 1986). Learned debate on the issues involved by scientists, doctors, lawyers, theologians, philosophers.

The Reproduction Revolution by Peter Singer and Deane Wells (Oxford University Press, 1984). The options so far available and unavailable to medics and prospective parents (the authors, incidentally, favour surrogate motherhood); plus an examination of the actual and potential ethical issues involved.

In the Name of Eugenics by Daniel J. Kevles (Penguin, 1986). The relationship between human genetics and the urge to improve human breeding stock – plus its inherent dangers.

Medical finance

Health Service Efficiency and Clinical Freedom (Folio No. 2) by Alan Williams (Nuffield Provincial Hospitals Trust, 1984). Outlines the grounds on which doctors make decisions. Professor Williams is professor of economics at York University; watch for his views on health care economics in the media.

Sex and health education

Health Education from Five to 16 (Curriculum matters No. 6); Her Majesty's Inspectors of Schools (HMSO, 1986). What should be done, by the topmost authorities on the British education curriculum.

General

Law and Morals: Warnock, Gillick and Beyond by Simon Lee (Oxford University Press, 1986). The main current debates on 'body ethics', plus proposals for keeping them under review, by a Catholic liberal.

Law and order by Adam Hopkins and Gaby Macphedran (Macdonald, 1985). The relationship between the individual and the state, as it is affected by law; for school/college students.

The Use of Drugs by Brian Ward (Macdonald, 1985). The ethical issues involved in the use of drugs; in the same series as *Law and Order*, and the present volume.

JOURNALS

Company Monthly magazine for women, published by the National Magazine Co Ltd. Invaluable on all questions of 'body ethics' for women, and some for men. Recent editions that are particularly useful are:
September, 1984; May, 1985; September, 1986 (the Pill)
January, 1986 (doctors' files)
October, 1986 (doctor-patient relationships)
February, 1987 (AIDS)

Health Education Journal Quarterly journal on health issues, published by the Health Education Authority.

The Independent Daily newspaper, published by Newspaper Publishing PLC. The weekly health page (Tuesdays) is outstanding.

Milbank Quarterly US quarterly, from the Milbank Foundation, 1 East 75th Street, New York, NY 10021. Vol 64, Supplement I is a special AIDS issue.

New Society Weekly journal, published by New Society Ltd. Essential reading: deals with all social aspects of late twentieth-century life ('body ethics' and medical care among them). Libraries often store it on file – use the index in each volume to browse. Especially useful recent editions are:

29 March, 1984 and 2 January, 1987 (medical finance)
7 February, 1985 (abortion)
30 August, 1985; 28 March and 5 September, 1986 (euthanasia)
7 March, 1986; 16 January 1987, (smoking statistics)
9 May, 1986 (embryo research and male pregnancy)
6 June, 1986 (blood transfusions)
15 August 1986, (abortion statistics)
29 August, 1986 (medical treatment of prisoners)
14 November, 1986 (AIDS)

The Times Daily newspaper, published by Times Newspapers Ltd. The features and letters column are particularly worth reading.

Useful addresses

Action on Smoking and Health (ASH) Ltd, 5–11 Mortimer Street, London W1.

Board of Deputies of British Jews, Woburn House, Upper Woburn Place, London WC1.

Catholic Marriage Advisory Council, 15 Lansdowne Road, London W11.

College of Health, 18 Victoria Park Square, London E2.

Church of England Board for Social Responsibility, Church House, Great Smith Street, London SW1.

Family Planning Information Service, 27 Mortimer Street, London W1.

Health Education Authority, 78 New Oxford Street, London WC1.

Islamic Cultural Centre and London Central Mosque, 146 Park Road, London NW8.

Jehovah's Witnesses, Watch Tower House, The Ridgeway, London NW7.

Life, 118–120 Warwick Street, Leamington Spa, Warwickshire CV32 4QW.

Medical Council on Alcoholism, 1 St Andrew's Place, London NW1

National Council for Christian Standards in Society, Whitehall House, 41 Whitehall, London SW1.

National Council for Civil Liberties, 21 Tabard Street, London SE1.

Religious Society of Friends (Quakers), Friends House, Euston Road, London NW1.

Road Safety Division, Royal Society for the Prevention of Accidents (RoSPA), Cannon House, Priory Queensway, Birmingham B4 6BS.

Society for the Protection of Unborn Children, 7 Tufton Street, London SW1.

Society of Teachers Opposed to Physical Punishment (STOPP), 18 Victoria Park, London E2.

Terrence Higgins Trust Ltd, BM AIDS, London WC1.

Voluntary Euthanasia Society, 13 Prince of Wales Terrace, London W8.

Credits

Age Concern England: 46b.
Associated Press: 43
Barnaby's Picture Library: 34, 49, 53.
BPCC/Aldus Archive: 6, 9b.
Camera Press: 14, 27, 29b, 36–37, 39, 59.
Robert Cappa/Magnum: 10.
Robert Cohen/AGIP: 22.
Anita Corbin/Format: 30.
Melanie Friend: 23.
Sally & Richard Greenhill: 35, 51, 52.
Paul Harrison/IPPF: 25.
Health Education Council: 18, 24.
The Independent: 54, 56 Jeremy Nicholl.
Keston College: 40.
Leicester Mercury: 41.
Barry Lewis/Network: front cover.
Library of Congress: 20.
MacQuitty International Collection: 46t.
Mansell Collection: 58.
Jenny Matthews/Format: 19.
Mercedes-Benz: 17r.
Hugh Olliff: 50.
Rex: 12t.
Science Photo Library: 7, 31, 32, 33.
STOPP: 9t.
Topham: 5, 12b, 15, 17l, 21, 38, 44, 48, 57.
Val Wilmer/Format: 29t.

In addition, the author would like to thank
Michael Pollard, Nicholas Pollard and RoSPA
for their help with the preparation of this book.

Index